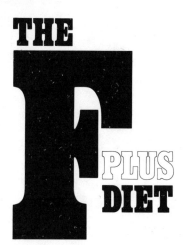

THE F PLUS DIET

THE F PLUS DIET

AUDREY EYTON

CROWN PUBLISHERS, INC.
NEW YORK

Introduction copyright © 1984 by Audrey Eyton
American edition copyright © 1985 by Crown Publishers, Inc., and Bantam Books, Inc.

British edition published in 1984 under the title *Audrey Eyton's Even Easier F-Plan* by Allen Lane, a division of Penguin Books, 536 Kings Road, London SW10 OUH, England.

Published in the United States by Crown Publishers, Inc., One Park Avenue, New York, New York 10016, and published in Canada by Bantam Books, Inc., 666 Fifth Avenue, New York, New York 10103.

CROWN is a trademark of Crown Publishers, Inc.

Manufactured in the United States of America

Library of Congress Cataloging in Publication Data

Eyton, Audrey.
   The F-plus diet.
   1. High-fiber diet—Recipes.   2. Low-calorie diet—Recipes.   I. Title.
   RM237.6.E98   1985   613.2'8   84-23841
   ISBN 0-517-55738-X

10 9 8 7 6 5 4 3 2 1

First American Edition

Contents

F-Plus—Now Even Easier!

You have already heard, or discovered for yourself, that the F-Plan is the easiest weight-loss method ever devised. Now you can be spoon-fed your daily dose of health-protecting, weight-loss-assisting dietary fiber.

How much dietary fiber should you consume in a day? Don't worry. Just follow any of the dozens of complete daily menus in this book and you will get the right amount of fiber from the correctly varied sources. How do you count the calories? Don't count—again, just follow the menus; the calories have already been counted for controlled weight loss.

The first F-Plan book, which made publishing history when it was released two years ago, offered a wide range of high-fiber low-calorie meals from which you could put together your own high-fiber weight-loss menus. Now this companion volume adds a new element of effortlessness. No need to add up or work out what you are going to eat. Just thumb through, pick out the type of menu that suits you best, and follow one each day.

Hate to cook? Haven't time to fuss? On pages 139–158 you'll find a wide range of F-Plan daily menus making maximum use of canned and packaged foods. Rushing off to work and wondering how to get an F-Plan diet lunch? The F-Plan menus with packed lunches starting on page 50 will be just right for you. Prefer to plan ahead and cook most of your F-Plan meals in advance? Sensible you. On page 224 you'll see how to do it, making maximum use of your freezer.

Whether man, woman, or child, you will find F-Plan full-day menus to suit you and your life-style in this book. We've done all the thinking and planning and putting it together for you so that all you need to do to get slim and fit is to make it (or buy it) and eat it. The F-Plan is easier than ever. Now it's up to you.

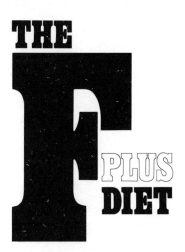

THE F PLUS DIET

Introduction

Except for those who have recently returned from a two-year expedition into the South American interior (in which case, living off the land, they have probably inadvertently been following it already!), the F-Plan diet needs little further introduction to the American public. In two years the name has become familiar to everybody. To compare its all-time record-breaking sale with that of any diet in the past would be similar to comparing the size of a baked potato with that of a baked bean.

Travel to the furthest ends of the earth and *The F-Plan* provides an instant topic of communication. Breathe its name, if you will, next time you visit Reykjavik and you will discover that there is an Icelandic edition. Travel to New Zealand and you will learn how it made history there—the fastest-selling book (fiction or nonfiction) in the publishing records of the country. In Australia it broke all diet-book sales records, in Canada it shot to the top of the best-seller lists within days of publication. In America, birthplace of all the previous diet-book blockbusters, it overcame initial skepticism—"A diet from *Britain?*"—by becoming the first imported diet to make the best-seller lists month after month. Even Islam has embraced it with an alcohol-free edition. It has become the best-selling diet in the world.

Now why on earth, literally, has the F-Plan caused such a fuss?

It is, understandably, in the nature of the overweight person to seek eagerly for the revolutionary new method that will provide an easier solution to that stubborn weight problem. It is in the nature of the diet-book writer to try to provide it. However, the diet-book writer of yesteryear labored under the difficulty of having to *invent* a "revolution"—a task that the fearless and the imaginative did not hesitate to tackle. As one leading

1

nutritionist remarked, plaintively, of a famous American best-selling diet of a few years ago: "I have no objection at all to its being at the top of the best-seller list. But why did they list it in the nonfiction rather than the fiction section?"

However, quietly, in the universities and research laboratories of the affluent world, a remarkable thing has been emerging over the past few years. A nutritional revolution, a *real* one. A major and almost complete about-turn in the beliefs about which foods we should eat more abundantly and which we should ration more stringently if we are concerned about losing weight and protecting our health.

To put it very simplistically, animal foods were in the recent past considered the outstanding source of most goodness, and animal protein acquired an almost magical aura of virtue. Lucky us, in the affluent world, to be able to indulge lavishly in meat and cream while the rest of the world had to struggle along on . . . well, peasant food like beans, root vegetables, and coarsely ground bread.

When struggling to reduce our weight, which somehow continued to increase on this regimen, we were urged to keep eating all that really valuable animal food and cut out the second-class foods that really didn't matter much: potatoes, bread, grains, and things of that ilk.

There was a snag. On our high-animal-food diets, we in the affluent world were getting fatter and fatter. We were also being killed off at an alarming rate by coronaries and illnesses like cancer of the colon that were hardly known in countries existing on a much higher proportion of cereal, fruit, and vegetable food. What we were eating, overabundantly, as an unavoidable part of our high-animal-food diet, was a large quantity of fat—and recent research has discovered close links between this high fat intake and both obesity and coronary heart disease. All animal foods, even the leaner meats, contain a significant amount of fat.

What we weren't eating was a seemingly unimportant substance found in those peasant foods like beans and unrefined cereals—dietary fiber. Again, recent research in nutrition has indicated that the importance of this substance has been vastly underestimated, in helping us both control our weight and protect our health against the major Western killer diseases.

Pity the poor dieter. Prior to the nutritional about-turn, he or she was being urged to eat many of the most fattening foods and to cut out the most helpful foods, like root vegetables, cereals, and bread, which would have been filling with a much lower intake of calories.

Pity the poor health enthusiast—chewing quantities of steak and swooshing down gallons of whole milk—and likely clogging up his or her arteries with coronary-inducing cholesterol.

It was no one's fault, really. Nutrition is a relatively new and inexact science in the early stages of discovery, and the leaders of the profession are now willing and anxious to say, albeit in their own language: "Look, folks, we got it wrong." They do so, for instance, in the 1983 Health Education Council publication, *A Discussion Paper on Proposals for Nutritional Guidelines for Health Education in Britain* (nutritionists were never strong on fun titles!), with this statement:

The previous nutritional advice in the UK to limit the intake of all carbohydrates as a means of weight control now runs counter to current thinking and contrary to the present proposals for a nutrition policy for the population as a whole. It is important, therefore, that a key feature of nutrition education should deal with counteracting the results of decades of teaching aimed at reducing carbohydrate intakes.

Which brings us right to the F-Plan. The F-Plan is a *high*-carbohydrate diet, rich in the beneficial fiber-rich carbohydrate foods: unrefined cereals, fruit, and vegetables. It is a low-fat diet. Most high-fiber foods are practically fat-free. At the same time, it moderates your intake of sugar. In fact, it incorporates all the new major nutritional guidelines for weight control and health, with the possible exception of salt reduction (an excess of salt is now widely considered to be a health hazard). You can reduce salt intake while following the F-Plan just as easily as on any other pattern of eating. The question of timing is left to you, simply because—realistically—those who attempt too many changes at once often find the task over-difficult. Give up smoking, lose that excess weight—but you will have a much greater chance of achieving both if you don't attempt the superhuman task of doing them both together. In the same way, the transitional period, during which you are concentrating on losing weight and getting used to eating less fat and more fiber, may not be the ideal time to sacrifice your salt as well. You may prefer to wait until F-Plan eating has become effortlessly familiar before tackling the salt issue.

The F-Plan is NEWtrition—made realistic. It does not flinch at the sight of a supermarket can or avoid a handily packaged slice of frozen haddock in favor of a rod and line. It is not for extremists. It is for normal people who would like to be thinner and would naturally prefer to protect themselves against the major health hazards if it is reasonably easy and practical to do so. The F-Plan—to the horror of the hair-shirt brigade—makes low-fat, high-fiber eating for weight control and health protection remarkably easy.

Prior to *The F-Plan* even health-conscious people aware of the increasing importance attached to dietary fiber intake found it difficult to know how to increase their intake sufficiently. Very few people knew which cereal, fruit, and vegetable foods were the richest sources of dietary fiber. You would need a good deal of expertise to extract this information from a nutrition textbook, in which the information would be given only in terms of percentage of dietary fiber per hundred grams. This is a far cry from knowing that there is a useful quantity in an apple (3.6 g), less in a stick of celery (0.3 g), and a surprisingly large quantity (6.7 g) in a small package of frozen peas.

Many people believed that increasing dietary fiber intake simply meant sprinkling a little bran on almost everything. Not only does this require a certain masochism—an eat-your-hair-shirt (rather than wearing it) mentality—but it rarely provides you with a sufficient quantity of the stuff. Neither, unlike the F-Plan, does it follow the primary dietary fiber rule for weight and health: Increase your intake from a wide range of foods— cereals, fruits, and vegetables.

The scientific research that has been reported during the two years since *The F-Plan* was published has added even more emphasis to the F-Plan method of obtaining dietary fiber from a range of foods rather than from any single source. Much remains to be discovered about the effects on weight and health of this highly complex substance, but it is known that dietary fiber obtained from different foods has different effects on the body. It would appear, for instance, that cereal fiber is particularly helpful in speeding the elimination processes, while if fiber plays a part, as some scientists suspect, in lowering cholesterol levels, it seems likely that the dietary fiber present in fruit is of particular value in this.

Because the F-Plan is based on scientific facts and steers its followers into adhering to today's major nutritional guidelines, it has been warmly welcomed and supported by leaders of the medical and nutritional world; many general practitioners today recommend it to their patients both as a weight-reducing diet and as a realistic method of increasing fiber intake for preventing or treating health problems. The author is particularly indebted to those great pioneers of dietary fiber research Dr. Dennis Burkitt and Dr. Hugh Trowell, who have been unfailingly generous in their encouragement and support. Not only that—by continuing to work with terrific energy in their seventies they add a splendid personal endorsement to their nutritional beliefs and fulfill the author's personal requirement of a good nutritionist: that he or she should live to a very ripe old age and finally have inscribed on his or her tombstone "I told you so!"

Of today's younger pioneers in this field of research, the author is particularly grateful to Dr. David Southgate, whose analytical principles form the foundation of the most widely used methods for measuring dietary fibers, and who has been most kind and supportive. Without Derek Miller, eminent research scientist and lecturer in nutrition at London University, there would probably have been no F-Plan; the author's debt to him, for many years of teaching and friendship, is immeasurable.

A second quiet revolution that has been going on over the past years is the realization, on the part of the leaders of the medical and nutritional professions, that there is a need to communicate nutrition guidelines to the public. No one has ever doubted the fact that the professional communicators of the media world are absolutely rotten at performing brain surgery. However, of late there has been increasing realization that a medical or scientific training is not necessarily ideal for learning the art of written communication. *The F-Plan*, which has measurably changed eating patterns in many parts of the world in a remarkably short time, is a happy example of how progress can be speeded when medical and scientific experts and communicators work happily hand in hand.

Of course, there have been a few critics. Those looking to find a flaw usually seize on the fact that in seeking to increase dietary fiber intake in a modern, realistic way the F-Plan makes use of handy prepackaged high-fiber foods like bran cereals and baked beans. And don't these—aha!—contain *sugar?*

Well yes, they do. And so do apples and pears and dates and grapes and lots of things made, not by Heinz or Crosse and Blackwell or Kellogg's, but by the Almighty. (It is always the policy of the author to turn for precedent to the very highest authority.)

In this age of excess weight in the Western world there can be no argument that we eat far too much sugar, which provides only calories—the things that make us fat—and none of the nutrients we need to keep our bodies functioning in a healthy way. Some nutritionists believe that our excessive intake of sugar contributes not only to obesity but to other health problems.

It is not the inclusion of sugar in our diets that causes these problems, but the inclusion of *enormous quantities* of sugar. In order to be thin and healthy we do not need to cut out all sugar; we need to cut out a good deal of sugar.

Which sugar? Well, it would seem reasonable that, for the sake of weight and health, we should first cut out those foods in which sugar is combined with nothing much that does us good and a good deal that does us harm. In many foods—chocolate, cookies, cakes, and ice cream—sugar is combined with fat, the most fattening of all foods, which we are also urged to restrict for the sake of our health. Obviously, sugar reduction should start with these doubly dangerous mega-baddies.

Next we come to foods and drinks that are more or less just plain or diluted sugar—sugar itself, sweet bottled and canned drinks, fat-free sweets like hard candy and mints, and (sorry, health-food enthusiasts) honey. Clearly these are the next candidates for curtailment.

Third, there is a category of foods in which sugar is combined with a good deal that is thought to do us good. An example of such a food is canned baked beans, in which sugar is used to add palatability to a rich source of vegetable protein, dietary fiber, and beneficial minerals and vitamins. Manufacturers: Heinz, Crosse and Blackwell, and Campbell.

Further examples are apples, pears, oranges, carrots, etc., in which sugar adds palatability to useful sources of dietary fiber and beneficial minerals and vitamins. Manufacturer: Mother Nature.

Recent research, in which babies during the first hours of their lives showed a gratified expression (no, not a burp) when a sugar solution was put on their tongues, suggests that our liking for sweetness is a natural, built-in predilection, not an acquired habit. It is the extraction of sugar from its natural sources, and so from its quantity-limiting association with dietary fiber, that would appear to be the root of the modern overconsumption problem.

When you follow the F-Plan you will consume considerably less sugar than you would on the average American diet, and the reduction will be mainly in the harmful (sugar-plus-fat) foods and the useless (sugar-plus-water) foods, rather than in those in which sugar is combined with dietary fiber and nutrients of value.

Talking of the burp, let us boldly mention a similar problem of greater social significance. To this criticism the F-Plan must openly plead guilty. If you switch from a low-fiber diet to one rich in vegetables . . . well, er, yes, it can indeed happen. Take comfort from the fact that it is largely a temporary adjustment problem, go easy on the beans, which are the main offenders at the start, and cheer yourself with the thought that, with millions of F-Plan enthusiasts worldwide, you are not alone with a flatulence problem.

These minor criticisms apart, it is somewhat difficult to criticize a diet that reverses all previous misconceptions about the most effective way to lose weight, provides a long-awaited, immeasurably better, new method, cuts down on the potentially harmful foods, and increases intake of health-protective food in direct accord with the new nutritional guidelines—and makes it all so *easy.*

With this book you will find the F-Plan even easier. Happy dieting and good health!

The Secret of the F-Plan

What the F-Plan does, which previous generations of weight-loss diets failed to do, is approximately double your intake of substances called dietary fiber as it reduces your calorie intake. Dietary fiber is essentially the cell-wall material of plants. It is present in all cereal foods, fruits, and vegetables, but some of these foods—whole-grain breads, bran cereals, strawberries, prunes, dates, peas, beans, and corn, for instance—have a particularly high content. The F-Plan makes use of fiber-rich foods to increase intake of dietary fiber from the 15–20 g a day usual in the American diet to 35–60 g daily.

The fact that a generous intake of dietary fiber is helpful to those attempting to lose surplus fat is unarguable. That is a very bold claim to make in the field of nutrition, where there are experts who will argue with almost anything. However, it is a claim that can be made with confidence, based on scientific evidence that either clearly proves or indicates that dietary fiber assists the dieter not just in one way but in a whole variety of ways.

Argue the weight of scientific evidence against any one slimming benefit, if you will, but you will still have to concede several other reasons why dieters should increase their intake of dietary fiber. Any one of these reasons would provide sufficient reason for following the high-fiber path to weight loss. What would be totally unarguable, in light of the research of recent years, would be the case for a *low*-fiber diet (like the once-popular low-carbohydrate diet) for dieting. To follow any diet that does not provide a generous quantity of fiber-rich foods is to deprive yourself of a range of benefits that start the moment the food goes into the mouth and continue right through the body to the final elimination process. These benefits have been revealed in detail in *The F-Plan*. However, here, for newcomers to the system, is a summary.

In the Mouth

High-fiber foods provide you with a large bulk of food for a moderate quantity of calories This, in itself, tends to lead to a lower calorie consumption—but there are additional benefits for dieters even before this food leaves the mouth. Fiber stimulates chewing, and scientific tests indicate that chewing promotes the sensation of satiety and fullness by a direct effect on the brain. The more you chew, the less you eat. Most overweight people eat considerably more quickly than thin people, and eating-behavior experts like psychiatrist Dr. Henry Jordan regard slower eating as one of the most vital factors in weight reduction. If its only effect were to slow your eating, as it undoubtedly does, a high-fiber diet would probably have a long-term effect in reducing your weight, but this is just the beginning of its benefits.

In the Stomach

High-fiber foods are the most filling foods of all. Dietary fiber is a spongelike substance that absorbs water and actually swells up in the stomach. The benefits for the dieter are obvious. On a high-fiber diet, as F-Plan dieters have discovered, you need never feel hungry, because not only is the food highly filling, it stays longer in the stomach than fiber-depleted food. When you are following a high-fiber diet you are taking a natural appetite suppressant as part of your food! Another reason why a high-fiber meal satisfies the appetite for longer than a typical Western fiber-depleted meal is associated with the blood sugar level. When blood sugar is low the body sends hunger signals to the brain, and this effect has been found to be particularly marked after meals based on low-fiber or fiber-free carbohydrate foods like sugar. However, a sufficient intake of dietary fiber solves this problem, adding a further long-term satiety bonus.

In the Elimination Process

Dietary fiber speeds the elimination of waste matter, which provides well-documented health benefits and may also be partly responsible for the increase in speed of weight loss that can be achieved on a high-fiber diet. In various scientific tests an examination of the feces of subjects on a high-fiber diet has shown them to contain more calories than is usual on a Westernized diet. One of the most recent tests, at London University's Department of Nutrition, indicates that this calorie waste can be as high as 20 percent on a high-fiber diet. This is a useful dieting bonus, since the less calories your body uses from food, the more it must draw from its own surplus fat. Clearly more research needs to be done in this area, but it is probable that some high-fiber foods will prove to be more effective in this than others.

Meanwhile, more scientific evidence is emerging pointing to yet another reason why F-Plan dieting is speedier as well as easier than other methods. Recent research indicates that on a high-carbohydrate diet—and the F-Plan is a high-carbohydrate low-fat diet—the metabolic rate, which is the rate at which you burn up calories, is faster than when you follow an animal-food-based high-fat diet.

If you consume 1,000 calories a day on the F-Plan, it seems that not only do some of them pass through undigested but also that the body may well be using up more calories than on other diets. So for your 1,000-calorie-a-day diet you could be achieving (at this stage of research one can only guess the figures) a weight loss that you would expect to achieve on 900 calories a day on any other diet.

Consider all the scientific facts and indications and what the F-Plan adds up to, quite simply, is this: more weight loss for less willpower.

No wonder it has become the world's best-selling diet.

Basic F-Plan Diet Rules

There are a few essential rules that you should follow whichever F-Plan diet variation you choose to suit your life-style. These rules and the reason for them are outlined here to help you follow your chosen diet.

1. Determine your total daily calorie intake, between a minimum of 1,000 and a maximum of 1,500 calories. See page 15 for guidance on your ideal dieting calorie total.

2. Aim at consuming daily between 35 g and 60 g of dietary fiber. This level of dietary fiber intake ensures that you will achieve the dieting benefits described in the Introduction. This has been made easy for you when you follow any of the diets, since each menu has been planned to provide between 35 g and 60 g of dietary fiber. If your normal diet is low in fiber, you may want to build up gradually to menus particularly rich in fiber.

3. Ensure that you reach your daily dietary fiber target from a variety of foods and that you consume some of the most essential nutrients for a healthy diet by eating certain foods daily. These foods are referred to as the "daily allowance" and are as follows:

• 1 cup of skim milk for adults and 2 cups for children
• 2 whole fresh fruits (an orange and an apple or pear)
• a daily portion of high-fiber cereal, usually Fiber-Filler (a type of homemade muesli). The ingredients and amounts are given on pages 13–14. Where this is not included in the daily allowance, an alternative packaged high-fiber breakfast cereal is included.

The total calorie and fiber counts for the daily-allowance foods are given at the top of each menu and do not appear in the individual meals.

12

4. Sugarless tea and coffee (artificial sweeteners can be used) and other drinks negligible in calories, such as water and low-calorie bottled and canned drinks, can be drunk at any time of day. No limit is set for these, but other drinks, especially alcoholic drinks, must be cut out or strictly limited if your diet is to succeed, since they can provide a large number of calories. See page 266 for further advice on alcoholic drinks.

Which of the following F-Plan diets you choose depends on your life-style—you may even decide that one diet suits you during the week and another on the weekends. So long as you choose a variety of menus for your daily calorie intake you will be following a healthy weight-reducing diet.

Fiber-Filler

Fiber-Filler has been specially devised to provide a useful portion of your daily dietary fiber from cereal, fruit, and nut sources. It has exceptional filling power and as such is a most valuable dieting aid. One daily portion of Fiber-Filler provides 15 g of dietary fiber and 220 calories.

To make your daily quantity of Fiber-Filler, mix together the following ingredients:

For 1 day

⅓ cup bran flakes
2 tablespoons bran
3 tablespoons Kellogg's Bran Buds
1 tablespoon slivered almonds
1 dried prune (chopped and pitted)
2 tablespoons (2 halves) chopped dried apricots
1 tablespoon raisins

If you find it easier to multiply the ingredients and make several daily servings at one time you can do so, but remember to mix the ingredients well since the bran tends to filter down to the bottom. To avoid this problem you could omit the bran and add 2 tablespoons of bran to each daily portion after dividing up.

For 8 days

2⅔ cups bran flakes
1   cup bran
1½ cups Kellogg's Bran Buds
½   cup chopped almonds
8   prunes, pitted and chopped
1   cup chopped dried apricots
½   cup raisins

Divide into daily quantities and package in separate plastic bags.

A Note on Supplements

Opinion is divided on whether those following a healthy weight-loss diet of varied food, like the F-Plan, would benefit from a nutrient supplement. Some nutritionists consider this unnecessary. Others argue that on a weight-losing 1,000 calories a day, half the average woman's usual food intake, there is a greater chance of being short of nutrients. Those sticking to this lower calorie level for more than two or three weeks may choose to take a daily multivitamin pill with iron to provide a useful safeguard during their weight-loss period.

A Note on Measurements

Standard teaspoons, tablespoons, and cups are used for these recipes. Unless otherwise indicated, a *level* spoon or cup should be used.

How Many Calories?

The F-Plan menus in this book provide 1,500 or 1,250 or 1,000 calories a day. *All* overweight people will lose weight on 1,000 calories daily—it is scientifically impossible not to do so. Most dieters will lose weight at the upper level of 1,500 calories daily. Here is a guide to help you choose the ideal level for you.

1,500-Calorie Menus
All men can lose weight on approximately 1,500 calories daily, but there is no reason why they should not follow the lower-calorie menus if they want a particularly rapid weight loss. Women who are more than 25 pounds overweight and are at the start of a dieting campaign can also usually lose weight quickly on approximately 1,500 calories daily, particularly if they are tall or of medium height.

1,250-Calorie Menus
Combining a good speed of weight loss with a reasonably ample diet, this is the ideal calorie intake for most women dieters.

1,000-Calorie Menus
Women who have particular difficulty losing weight at a satisfactory speed are recommended to keep to this lower level of calorie intake. Those most likely to come within this category are:

    1. Those who are only a few pounds overweight.
    2. Those who have already lost a good deal of weight and are in the later stages of a dieting campaign.
    3. Small women.

Mixing Menus

Weight loss depends on average calorie intake over a period of time, rather than on precise daily calorie intake, so many dieters might find it a good plan to mix 1,500-, 1,250-, and 1,000-calorie menus throughout the week to fit in with their own pattern of life. For instance, if you find, as many dieters do, that you can be stricter during the week than on weekends, you might follow 1,000-calorie menus from Monday to Friday and then switch to 1,500-calorie menus on Saturday and Sunday. On this pattern you would achieve the same weekly weight loss as you would on approximately 1,150 calories daily. On this averaging-out basis, there is no reason why most dieters cannot freely draw on any diet menu in this book.

The menus in this section provide the types of meals that have proved most popular with F-Plan dieters: plenty of nice ideas but never too much fuss or effort in shopping or cooking. The menus all follow the basic F-Plan rules (see page 12) and are divided into three meals a day, plus a snack. All the meals are quick and simple to prepare, and the foods are readily available.

The section is divided up into two parts: approximately 1,000 calories and 1,250 calories daily, all providing 35–60 g fiber. They are designed for fast weight loss with the minimum of fuss.

Special Diet Notes

1. Begin by deciding which daily calorie total will give you a satisfactory weight loss. You will find guidance on page 15.

2. Select the menus from those of your chosen daily calorie total for one week at a time so that you can plan the shopping and always have the right foods available.

3. Vary the menus chosen to ensure that you eat a wide variety of foods.

4. Do *not* swap individual meals from one menu to another, since all the menus have been carefully calculated for a full day.

5. Make up the Fiber-Filler for your daily allowance either daily or for several days in one batch, following the recipe on page 13.

6. Allow yourself as much tea and coffee *without sugar* (sweeteners can be used) as you wish throughout the day *so long as* you use only the skim milk that remains from your daily allowance after you have had your Fiber-Filler. In addition, you can drink as much water and drinks labeled "low-calorie" as you wish. Alcoholic drinks are not included in these menus; however, should you feel the need for an occa-

sional alcoholic drink, see the advice on alcoholic drinks on page 266.

1,000-Calorie Menu #1

	Calories	Fiber (g)
Daily allowance: Fiber-Filler, 1 cup skim milk, an orange, and an apple or pear	450	23.0
Breakfast Half portion of Fiber-Filler with milk from allowance		
Lunch *Pizza Toasts Orange from allowance	381	7.2
Evening meal 4 ounces frozen cod cooked in 1 teaspoon low-cal margarine ¾ cup fresh or frozen peas, boiled ¾ cup carrots, boiled Apple or pear from allowance	223	10.7
Snack Remaining Fiber-Filler with milk from allowance		
Total	**1,054**	**40.9**

*PIZZA TOASTS   *Serves 1*

2   large thin slices of whole-grain bread (Pepperidge Farm Honey Wheatberry)
2   small tomatoes, sliced

*Throughout the book an asterisk indicates that the recipe follows for this particular dish.

Salt and pepper to taste
¼ teaspoon dried thyme or mixed herbs
½ cup grated mozzarella cheese
2 ripe olives, sliced

Toast the bread on both sides. Cover both slices of toast with the tomatoes. Season well and sprinkle on the herbs. Top with grated cheese and garnish with olive slices. Grill until the cheese is melted. Serve hot.

1,000-Calorie Menu #2

	Calories	Fiber (g)
Daily allowance: Fiber-Filler, 1 cup skim milk, an orange, and an apple or pear	450	23.0

Breakfast
Half portion of Fiber-Filler with milk from allowance
Orange from allowance

Lunch

⅔ cup cottage cheese (plain, with chives, with onion and peppers, or with pineapple) served with ½ cup diced, cooked, and drained beets mixed with 5 mushrooms (sliced), 1 large celery stalk (finely chopped), and 2 tablespoons oil-free French dressing		
A few sprigs of parsley		
Apple or pear from allowance	196	4.2

Evening meal
* Baked Potato and Beef

1 cup shredded white cabbage, tossed with 1 tablespoon oil-free French dressing	303	8.0

Snack
Remaining Fiber-Filler with milk from
   allowance

Total	**949**	**35.2**

*BAKED POTATO WITH BEEF   *Serves 1*

1	large baking potato
3	ounces ground beef
1	small onion, chopped
½	cup drained and chopped canned tomatoes plus ¼ cup reserved juice
	Dash of Worcestershire sauce
	Salt and pepper to taste
1	heaping tablespoon frozen peas

Scrub the potato well, then bake by one of the following methods:

1. Put the potato in the center of a moderately hot oven (400°F) for 45 minutes, or until soft when pricked with a fork.

2. Put the potato in a pan of water, bring to a boil, then simmer gently for 20 minutes. Drain. Bake the potato in a moderately hot oven (375°F) for 10 to 15 minutes to crisp the skin.

3. Prick well all over and cook in a microwave oven on full power for 4 minutes, turning after 2 minutes.

Meanwhile, put the ground beef, onion, tomatoes, and tomato juice in a small pan. Add the Worcestershire sauce and salt and pepper. Heat to a boil, cover, and simmer gently for 15 minutes. Stir in the peas and heat through. Cut the baked potato in half lengthwise and scoop out some of the flesh. Mix it with the hot beef mixture and pile back into the potato jacket.

1,000-Calorie Menu #3

	Calories	Fiber (g)
Daily allowance: Fiber-Filler, 1 cup skim milk, an orange, and an apple or pear	450	23
Breakfast Half portion of Fiber-Filler with milk from allowance		
Lunch *Kidney Bean Soup 1 large thin slice of Pepperidge Farm Honey Wheatberry bread Apple or pear from allowance	193	12
Evening meal *Cheese and Corn Omelet 1 medium tomato, raw or grilled without fat ½ cup plain low-fat yogurt with orange from allowance and artificial sweetener, if necessary	328	6
Snack Remaining Fiber-Filler with milk from allowance		
Total	**971**	**41**

*KIDNEY BEAN SOUP   *Serves 1*

½   cup canned kidney beans, drained
3   tablespoons chopped onion
1   large celery stalk, chopped
1   cup beef bouillon

1   bay leaf
     Salt and pepper to taste
¼   teaspoon chili powder

Put all the ingredients in a saucepan. Bring to a boil, cover, and simmer for 30 minutes. Remove the bay leaf and serve the soup as is, or purée in a blender if preferred.

*CHEESE AND CORN OMELET   *Serves 1*

1   egg
2   tablespoons water
     Salt and pepper to taste
     Dash of Worcestershire sauce
1   teaspoon diet margarine
½   cup canned corn, drained
2   tablespoons green pepper, finely chopped
¼   cup grated Cheddar cheese

Beat together the egg, water, salt and pepper, and Worcestershire sauce. Grease a nonstick omelet pan with margarine and heat. Pour in the egg and cook gently until almost set. Sprinkle on the corn, green pepper, and grated cheese. Heat under the broiler until the cheese begins to melt. Fold the omelet and serve.

1,000-Calorie Menu #4

	Calories	Fiber (g)
Daily allowance: Fiber-Filler, 1 cup skim milk, an orange, and an apple or pear	450	23.0
Breakfast Half portion of Fiber-Filler with milk from allowance		

Lunch
¾ cup canned baked beans in tomato
    sauce, heated, served on 1 large thin
    slice of Pepperidge Farm Honey
    Wheatberry bread, toasted; garnish
    with 1 medium tomato, cut into
    wedges

Orange from allowance	346	27.4

Evening meal
1 (3-ounce) slice of cooked fresh ham
½ cup canned peas
½ cup Brussels sprouts, boiled

¼ cup vanilla ice cream	284	7.5

Snack
Remaining Fiber-Filler with milk from
    allowance
Apple or pear from allowance

Total	**1,080**	**57.9**

1,000-Calorie Menu #5

	Calories	Fiber (g)
Daily allowance: Fiber-Filler, 1 cup skim milk, an orange, and an apple or pear	450	23.0

Breakfast
Half portion of Fiber-Filler with milk
    from allowance
Orange from allowance

Lunch
*Tuna Salad Sandwich

Apple or pear from allowance	270	5.3

Evening meal
1 chicken leg and thigh (3½ ounces),
    skin removed, broiled
1 large potato, baked in its jacket, with
    1 tablespoon oil-free French dressing
2 tablespoons fresh or frozen peas   335   8.0

Snack
Remaining Fiber-Filler with milk from
    allowance

	Total	**1,055**	**36.3**

*TUNA SALAD SANDWICH   *Serves 1*

2   large thin slices of whole-wheat bread
1   tablespoon low-calorie salad dressing
¼   cup flaked water-packed tuna
1   lettuce leaf
1   tomato, sliced
½   medium cucumber, sliced

Spread both slices of bread with salad dressing and fill with the
remaining ingredients.

1,000-Calorie Menu #6

	Calories	Fiber (g)
Daily allowance: Fiber-Filler, 1 cup skim milk, an orange, and an apple or pear	450	23.0

Breakfast
Half-portion of Fiber-Filler with milk
    from allowance
Orange from allowance

Lunch
4 whole-wheat crackers (Wheat Thins),
   topped with ⅓ cup cottage cheese
   mixed with 2 chopped dates and 2
   tablespoons chopped walnuts
1 large celery stalk, cut into pieces
Apple or pear from allowance   241   3.4

Evening meal
* Egg Florentine
*Poached Citrus Plums   225   10.1

Snack
Remaining Fiber-Filler with milk from
   allowance

	Total	**916**	**36.5**

*EGG FLORENTINE   *Serves 1*

¾   cup frozen chopped spinach, thawed
1   egg
¼   cup plain low-fat yogurt
¼   teaspoon prepared mustard
    Salt and pepper to taste
2   tablespoons grated Cheddar cheese
3   tablespoons whole-wheat bread crumbs

Heat the spinach gently (without adding butter) in a small pan
or in a microwave oven, then spoon into a small fireproof dish.
Poach the egg and place on top of the spinach. Blend the
yogurt with the mustard and seasoning and spoon over the egg.
Mix the grated cheese and bread crumbs and sprinkle over the
top. Broil until the topping is crisp and brown.

*POACHED CITRUS PLUMS   *Serves 1*

2	medium-size fresh plums
¼	cup fresh orange juice
1	teaspoon sugar (optional)
2	teaspoons slivered almonds

Wash the plums and put them in a pan with the orange juice. Cover with a tight-fitting lid and heat gently for 5 minutes. Add the sugar. Serve hot or cold, sprinkled with the slivered almonds.

1,000-Calorie Menu #7

	Calories	Fiber (g)
Daily allowance: Fiber-Filler, 1 cup skim milk, an orange, and an apple or pear	450	23.0
Breakfast Half portion of Fiber-Filler with milk from allowance Orange from allowance		
Lunch *Lentil and Vegetable Soup 4 whole-wheat crackers (Wheat Thins) Apple or pear from allowance	124	5.3
Evening meal 3 (1-ounce) slices of lean boiled ham *Coleslaw 1 medium tomato, sliced ½ medium cucumber, sliced A few lettuce leaves		

1 large thin slice of Pepperidge Farm
   whole-wheat bread, spread with 1
   teaspoon margarine
25 green grapes   432   9.5

Snack
Remaining Fiber-Filler with milk from
   allowance

Total	**1,006**	**37.8**

*LENTIL AND VEGETABLE SOUP   *Serves 1*
(Several portions can be made at one time and frozen until
required.)

⅓   cup cooked and drained lentils
3   tablespoons chopped onion
1   medium carrot, sliced
1   large celery stalk, chopped
1   chicken bouillon cube dissolved in 1½ cups boiling water
     Salt and pepper to taste

Put all the ingredients in a pan. Bring to a boil, cover, and
simmer gently for 1 hour.

*COLESLAW   *Serves 1*

1   cup shredded cabbage
1   tablespoon finely chopped onion
1   small carrot, grated
1   tablespoon oil-free French dressing

Mix together the cabbage, onion, and carrot. Add the dressing
and toss well.

1,000-Calorie Menu #8

	Calories	Fiber (g)
Daily allowance: Fiber-Filler, 1 cup skim milk, an orange, and an apple or pear	450	23.0
Breakfast Half portion of Fiber-Filler with milk from allowance		
Lunch *Crunchy Sardine Sandwich Apple or pear from allowance	284	5.6
Evening meal *Baked Potato with Chicken Liver Filling ¼ cup green beans, boiled Orange from allowance	327	9.0
Snack Remaining Fiber-Filler with milk from allowance		
Total	**1,061**	**37.6**

*CRUNCHY SARDINE SANDWICH   *Serves 1*

2   large thin slices of Pepperidge Farm whole-wheat bread
1   tablespoon low-calorie salad dressing
1   sardine in tomato sauce
1   cup fresh bean sprouts
1   tablespoon chopped green pepper

Spread the bread with salad dressing. Mash the sardine and spread on one slice of bread. Top with bean sprouts and green pepper and the second slice of bread. Cut into four sandwiches.

*BAKED POTATO WITH CHICKEN LIVER FILLING
Serves 1

1   large baking potato
3½ ounces chicken livers, chopped
3   tablespoons finely chopped onion
¼   cup corn
¼   cup water
    Salt and pepper to taste
1   teaspoon tomato purée

Bake the potato following one of the methods on page 20. Put the chicken livers, onion, corn, and water in a small pan. Add the salt and pepper and tomato purée. Heat to a simmer, cover, and simmer gently for 5 minutes. Cut the potato in half lengthwise and scoop out some of the flesh. Mix with the chicken liver mixture and pile back into the potato jacket. Serve at once.

1,000-Calorie Menu #9

	Calories	Fiber (g)
Daily allowance: Fiber-Filler, 1 cup skim milk, an orange, and an apple or pear	450	23.0

Breakfast
Half portion of Fiber-Filler with milk
from allowance

Lunch
*Mushroom and Tomato Scramble on
   Toast
Orange from allowance   297   5.5

Evening meal
3½ ounces cod or haddock fillets,
   brushed with 1 teaspoon diet
   margarine, broiled
¾ cup peas, boiled
½ cup canned tomatoes
½ banana   347   10.7

Snack
Remaining Fiber-Filler with milk from
   allowance
Apple from allowance

                           Total   1,094   39.2

*MUSHROOM AND TOMATO SCRAMBLE ON TOAST
   Serves 1

2   large thin slices of bran bread
¼   cup skim milk (in addition to allowance)
5   small mushrooms, sliced
1   egg
     Salt and pepper to taste
1   medium tomato, chopped
1   tablespoon chopped parsley (optional)

Toast the bread. Put the milk and mushrooms in a pan. Heat
gently for 3 minutes. Beat the egg with salt and pepper and stir
into the mushrooms. Cook, stirring continuously, until the egg
is creamy. Stir in the chopped tomato. Top the two slices of
toast with the mushroom and tomato scramble. Sprinkle with
chopped parsley.

1,000-Calorie Menu #10

	Calories	Fiber (g)
Daily allowance: Fiber-Filler, 1 cup skim milk, an orange, and an apple or pear	450	2.30
Breakfast Half portion of Fiber-Filler with milk from allowance Orange from allowance		
Lunch *Creamy Spinach Soup 4 whole wheat crackers Apple or pear from allowance	183	10.7
Evening meal *Savory Beef 2 tablespoons instant mashed potatoes (no butter) 12 Brussels sprouts, boiled ⅓ cup blueberries 1 medium apple, peeled, cored, and sliced 2 tablespoons water and 1½ teaspoons sugar	432	13.0
Snack Remaining Fiber-Filler with milk from allowance		
Total	**1,065**	**46.7**

*CREAMY SPINACH SOUP   *Serves 1*
(Several portions can be made up at one time and frozen until required.)

¾   cup frozen chopped spinach, thawed
1   cup skim milk
1   tablespoon instant oatmeal
     Salt and pepper to taste
     Grated nutmeg to taste

Put the spinach, milk, and oatmeal in a pan. Bring to a boil and simmer for 3 minutes. Purée in a blender and season with salt and pepper and nutmeg.

*SAVORY BEEF   *Serves 1*

4   ounces lean ground beef
1   small onion, finely chopped
1   celery stalk, finely chopped
¼   cup beef bouillon
     Salt and pepper to taste
     Pinch of mixed herbs
1   teaspoon tomato purée
1   tablespoon frozen peas

Fry the beef in a nonstick saucepan until well browned. Drain off all the fat that runs out of the meat. Add the onion, celery, and bouillon to the meat in the pan and bring to a boil, stirring. Reduce the heat, season with salt and pepper, add the herbs and tomato purée, and stir. Cover and simmer for 30 minutes, stirring occasionally and adding more water if needed. Stir in the peas and heat through for 5 minutes.

1,250-Calorie Menu #1

	Calories	Fiber (g)
Daily allowance: Fiber-Filler, 1 cup skim milk, an orange, and an apple or pear	450	23.0
Breakfast Half portion of Fiber-Filler with milk from allowance 1 large thin slice of bran bread, spread with 1 teaspoon diet margarine and 1 teaspoon honey or marmalade	114	2.6
Lunch *Corned Beef and Baked Bean Sandwich 1 small carrot stick Apple or pear from allowance	274	9.2
Evening meal *Ham and Pepper Omelet ⅔ cup mixed vegetables, boiled 1 cup juice-packed sliced peaches ¼ cup vanilla ice cream	455	10.0
Snack Remaining Fiber-Filler with milk from allowance Orange from allowance		
Total	**1,293**	**44.8**

*CORNED BEEF AND BAKED BEAN SANDWICH
Serves 1

2   large thin slices of bran bread
1   tablespoon tomato sauce
1   slice of canned corned beef
2   tablespoons canned baked beans in tomato sauce
     Pepper to taste
     A few slices of cucumber

Spread one slice of bread with tomato sauce. Mash the corned beef with the baked beans and pepper. Spread over one slice of the bread. Top with cucumber slices and cover with the second slice of bread.

*HAM AND PEPPER OMELET   *Serves 1*

1   egg
1   tablespoon water
     Salt and pepper to taste
1   teaspoon diet margarine
2   slices of lean boiled ham, chopped
½   small green pepper, chopped

Beat the egg with water and salt and pepper. Grease a nonstick omelet pan with margarine and heat. Pour in the egg mixture and cook gently until almost set. Sprinkle on the chopped ham and green pepper and heat under the broiler for 1 minute. Fold the omelet.

1,250-Calorie Menu #2

	Calories	Fiber (g)
Daily allowance: Fiber-Filler, 1 cup skim milk, an orange, and an apple or pear	450	23.0
Breakfast Half portion of Fiber-Filler with milk from allowance 1 large thin slice of whole-wheat bread, toasted and spread with 1 teaspoon dict margarine	94	1.2
Lunch 4 wheat crackers (Wheat Thins) spread with 2 tablespoons peanut butter and topped with 1 tomato (sliced), and ½ medium cucumber (sliced), and chopped lettuce 1 banana	252	5.8
Evening meal *Bologna Salad ⅔ cup fruit-flavored low-fat yogurt (blueberry, strawberry, cherry, etc.) Apple or pear from allowance	511	19.0
Snack Remaining Fiber-Filler with milk from allowance Orange from allowance		
Total	**1,307**	**49**

* BOLOGNA SALAD   *Serves 1*

¾   cup lima beans, cooked
1   slice of bologna, diced
1   small green pepper, chopped
2   radishes, sliced
2   to 3 scallions, chopped
2   tablespoons oil-free French dressing
    A few lettuce leaves

Put the lima beans, bologna, green pepper, radishes, and scallions in a bowl. Add the French dressing and toss well. Serve on a bed of lettuce leaves.

1,250-Calorie Menu #3

	Calories	Fiber (g)
Daily allowance: Fiber-Filler, 1 cup skim milk, an orange, and an apple or pear	450	23.0
Breakfast Half portion of Fiber-Filler with milk from allowance		
Lunch * Bean and Ham Toppers Orange from allowance	456	24.4
Evening meal * Macaroni and Cheese 25 green grapes	380	3.6

Snack
Remaining Fiber-Filler with milk from
  allowance
Apple or pear from allowance

Total	**1,286**	**51.0**

*BEAN AND HAM TOPPERS *Serves 1*

1   whole-wheat bagel
¼   teaspoon prepared mustard
¾   cup canned baked beans in tomato sauce
1   slice of lean boiled ham, chopped

Split the bagel and spread both halves with mustard. Heat the baked beans and pile on top. Sprinkle the chopped ham over the beans and serve.

*MACARONI AND CHEESE *Serves 1*

⅓   cup whole-wheat macaroni
1   tablespoon whole-wheat flour
⅓   cup skim milk (in addition to allowance)
1   teaspoon diet margarine
    Salt and pepper to taste
¼   teaspoon prepared mustard
3   tablespoons grated Cheddar cheese
1   medium tomato, sliced

Boil the macaroni in salted water for 12 minutes, or until tender; drain. Put the flour, milk, and margarine in a saucepan and heat, stirring continuously, until it boils and thickens. Season with salt and pepper. Add the mustard and cheese. Stir the macaroni into the sauce. Pour into an ovenproof dish. Top with tomato slices. Bake at 350° F for 20 minutes.

1,250-Calorie Menu #4

	Calories	Fiber (g)
Daily allowance: Fiber-Filler, 1 cup skim milk, an orange, and an apple or pear	450	23.0
Breakfast Half portion of Fiber-Filler with milk from allowance		
Lunch *Mushrooms and Corn on Toast 1 Granola Cluster (Quaker Oats Honey 'n Oats) Apple or pear from allowance	334	7.8
Evening meal *Sardine Salad 1 large baked potato (see page 20 for baking instructions), topped with 2 tablespoons low-fat yogurt mixed with 1 teaspoon tomato purée and salt and pepper to taste Orange from allowance	481	12.0
Snack Remaining Fiber-Filler with milk from allowance		
Total	**1,265**	**42.8**

*MUSHROOMS AND CORN ON TOAST   *Serves 1*

1   large slice of Pepperidge Farm whole-wheat bread
2   teaspoons cornstarch
½   cup skim milk (in addition to allowance)
⅓   cup canned button mushrooms
1   tablespoon low-fat yogurt
⅓   cup canned corn
    Salt and pepper to taste
    Dash of Worcestershire sauce

Toast the bread. Blend the cornstarch with the milk and stir in the mushrooms. Bring to a boil, stirring, and cook for 2 minutes, until thickened. Add the yogurt and corn. Season with salt and pepper and stir in the Worcestershire sauce. Serve on the toast.

*SARDINE SALAD   *Serves 1*

1½   large canned sardines in tomato sauce
     A few lettuce leaves
2   large celery stalks, chopped
⅔   cup grated carrot
2   heaping tablespoons fresh garden peas or thawed frozen
     peas
1   tablespoon oil-free French dressing

Arrange the sardines on the lettuce leaves. Mix the celery, carrot, and peas with the French dressing and serve with the sardines.

1,250-Calorie Menu #5

	Calories	Fiber (g)
Daily allowance: Fiber-Filler, 1 cup skim milk, an orange, and an apple or pear	450	23.0
Breakfast Half portion of Fiber-Filler with milk from allowance		
1 large slice of whole-wheat bread, toasted and spread with 1 teaspoon diet margarine and 2 teaspoons honey or marmalade	152	1.4
Lunch 1 hard-boiled egg served with a few lettuce leaves, 1 small grated carrot mixed with 1 tablespoon raisins, a few radishes, 3 tablespoons scallions, and 1 tablespoon low-calorie salad dressing		
½ cup fruit-flavored low-fat yogurt	344	6.7
Evening meal *Grilled Lamb Chop with Savory Topping		
¾ cup fresh or frozen peas, cooked		
1 large carrot, boiled		
Orange from allowance	344	12.4
Snack Remaining Fiber-Filler with milk from allowance		
Apple or pear from allowance		
Total	**1,290**	**43.5**

*GRILLED LAMB CHOP WITH SAVORY TOPPING
Serves 1

1 (5-ounce) loin lamb chop
1 small onion, sliced
½ cup chopped canned tomatoes
  Dash of Worcestershire sauce
  Salt and pepper to taste
1 tablespoon whole-wheat bread crumbs
  Generous pinch of dried mixed herbs

Broil the lamb chop. Meanwhile, heat the sliced onion, tomatoes, Worcestershire sauce, and salt and pepper in a pan for
5 minutes, or until the onion is softened. Put half the onion and
tomato mixture in a small heatproof dish. Put the grilled lamb
chop on top and spoon on the remaining onion and tomato
mixture. Mix the bread crumbs with the herbs and sprinkle
evenly over the chop. Broil until bread crumbs are crisp and
browned.

1,250-Calorie Menu #6

	Calories	Fiber (g)
Daily allowance: Fiber-Filler, 1 cup skim milk, an orange, and an apple or pear	450	23.0
Breakfast Half portion of Fiber-Filler with milk from allowance 1 Ryvita crispbread, spread with 1 teaspoon honey or marmalade	59	1.0
Lunch *Crunchy Salad with Ham 2 Ryvita crispbreads, spread with 1 teaspoon diet margarine Orange from allowance	381	8.0

Evening meal
2 canned pork dinner sausages, grilled
1 medium-size tomato, halved, grilled
   without fat
½ cup canned baked beans in tomato
   sauce
1 medium boiled potato, mashed using
   skim milk from allowance and no
   butter, or 2 tablespoons instant
   mashed potatoes, made up without
   butter   397   15.25

Snack
Remaining Fiber-Filler with milk from
   allowance
Apple or pear from allowance

	Total	**1,287**	**47.25**

CRUNCHY SALAD WITH HAM   *Serves 1*

1   cup shredded red cabbage
1   carrot, grated
1   small onion, thinly sliced
1   tablespoon oil-free French dressing
1   tablespoon diet mayonnaise
2   (1-ounce) slices of lean boiled ham

Mix together the cabbage, carrot, and onion. Add the French dressing and mayonnaise and toss until thoroughly blended. Serve with the slices of ham.

1,250-Calorie Menu #7

	Calories	Fiber (g)
Daily allowance: Fiber-Filler, 1 cup skim milk, an orange, and an apple or pear	450	23.0
Breakfast Half portion of Fiber-Filler with milk from allowance		
1 egg, poached and served on 1 large slice of whole-wheat bread, toast	156	1.2
Lunch *Cauliflower Soup		
4 wheat crackers (Wheat Thins), spread with 1 teaspoon diet margarine		
1 apple or pear from allowance	134	4.3
Evening meal 4 (1-ounce) slices of Canadian bacon, grilled, served with 2 juice-packed pineapple rings, grilled		
½ cup corn		
½ cup green beans		
4 whole-wheat crackers served with ¼ cup mozzarella cheese and 1 large celery stalk	584	10.3
Snack Remaining Fiber-Filler with milk from allowance		
Orange from allowance		
Total	**1,324**	**38.8**

*CAULIFLOWER SOUP   *Serves 1*

1½ cups cauliflower florets
1   small onion, chopped
1   cup chicken bouillon
1   tablespoon nonfat dry milk powder
     Salt and pepper to taste
2   teaspoons grated Parmesan cheese

Put the cauliflower and onion in a small saucepan and add chicken bouillon. Cook until the vegetables are tender, about 15 to 20 minutes. Purée the soup in a blender. Return to the pan. Beat in the milk and season with salt and pepper. Reheat gently. Serve topped with the Parmesan cheese.

1,250-Calorie Menu #8

	Calories	Fiber (g)
This menu is suitable for vegetarians.		
Daily allowance: Fiber-Filler, 1 cup skim milk, an orange, and an apple or pear	450	23.0
Breakfast Half portion of Fiber-Filler with milk from allowance		
1 egg, boiled and served with 1 Ryvita crispbread, spread with 1 teaspoon diet margarine	134	1.0
Lunch 1 whole-wheat English muffin, split, toasted, and filled with 2 tablespoons peanut butter		
⅔ cup grated carrot, and 1 lettuce leaf Orange from allowance	368	9.5

Evening meal
*Ratatouille au Gratin
¾ cup fresh or frozen raw raspberries or
   strawberries   362   24.7
                              with berries
Or
¼ cup vanilla ice cream   377   17.3
                           with ice cream

Snack
Remaining Fiber-Filler with milk from
   allowance
Apple from allowance

Total   with berries 1,314   58.2

with ice cream 1,329   50.8

*RATATOUILLE AU GRATIN   *Serves 1*

1   small eggplant (1 cup diced or 6 slices)
     Salt and pepper to taste
1   medium onion, peeled and sliced
1   cup diced or sliced zucchini
2   medium tomatoes, sliced
¼   teaspoon dried basil
¼   teaspoon dried oregano
¼   cup grated Muenster cheese
1   large slice of Pepperidge Farm whole-wheat bread

Cut the eggplant into ¼-inch slices. Sprinkle the cut surfaces
with salt, then let stand for 30 minutes to draw out the juices.
Rinse the eggplant, drain, and dry. Put eggplant slices, onion,
zucchini, tomatoes, and herbs in an ovenproof dish. Season
with salt and pepper. Sprinkle the grated cheese on top. Bake
at 350° F for 30 minutes, until the vegetables are tender. Serve
with the bread to mop up the juices.

1,250-Calorie Menu #9

	Calories	Fiber (g)
This menu is suitable for vegetarians.		
Daily allowance: Fiber-Filler, 1 cup skim milk, an orange, and an apple or pear	450	23.0
Breakfast Half portion of Fiber-Filler with milk from allowance ½ banana	43	1.4
Lunch *Cheese and Apple Sandwich ¼ cup fruit-flavored low-fat yogurt	377	3.5
Evening meal *Layered Bean Casserole Orange from allowance	392	33.0
Snack Remaining Fiber-Filler with milk from allowance 1 cup chocolate milk: 1 teaspoon chocolate syrup and ¾ cup skim milk (in addition to allowance)	85	0.0
Total	**1,347**	**60.9**

*CHEESE AND APPLE SANDWICH   *Serves 1*

1   tablespoon diet mayonnaise
¼   cup grated Swiss cheese
2   large slices of Pepperidge Farm Honey Wheatberry bread
     Apple from allowance

Mix mayonnaise with grated cheese and spread over both slices of bread. Cut the apple in half. Core one half and slice thinly. Arrange the apple slices over one of the cheese-covered slices of bread and top with the second slice of bread. Cut the remaining half apple into wedges and eat with the sandwich.

*LAYERED BEAN CASSEROLE   *Serves 1*

⅓   cup canned kidney beans, drained
½   cup canned lima beans, drained
¾   cup chopped canned tomatoes
3   tablespoons finely chopped onion
     Salt and pepper to taste
     Pinch of dried basil
¾   cup cooked frozen chopped spinach, drained
     Grated nutmeg
1   small (¾-ounce) package of potato chips, crushed

Spoon the kidney beans into a small ovenproof casserole. Cover with the lima beans. Mix the tomatoes with the onion, salt and pepper, and basil, and spoon over the beans. Spread the spinach on top and sprinkle on a little grated nutmeg. Cover and bake at 375° F for 35 minutes. Uncover and sprinkle on the crushed potato chips. Return to the oven for 5 minutes, uncovered.

1,250-Calorie Menu #10

	Calories	Fiber (g)
This menu is suitable for vegetarians.		
Daily allowance: Fiber-Filler, 1 cup skim milk, an orange, and an apple or pear	450	23.0
Breakfast Whole portion of Fiber-Filler with milk from allowance		
Lunch 1 cup canned spaghetti in tomato sauce, heated and covered with 1 sliced tomato and 1 tablespoon grated Parmesan cheese Apple or pear from allowance	224	2.6
Evening meal *Vegetable Paella Fruit salad made with 1 small bunch of grapes, orange from allowance (segmented), 1 medium banana (sliced), and ¼ cup apple juice	507	16.5
Snack ½ cup low-fat yogurt with 2 teaspoons honey	90	0.0
Total	**1,271**	**42.1**

*VEGETABLE PAELLA *Serves 1*

2   tablespoons raw brown rice
1   small onion, chopped
1   small green pepper, chopped
2   tomatoes, chopped
5   small mushrooms, sliced
1   heaping tablespoon fresh or frozen peas
¼   teaspoon dried thyme or marjoram
¼   teaspoon grated lemon rind
    Salt and pepper to taste
2   tablespoons roasted peanuts or cashew nuts (15 nuts)

Put the rice, onion, green pepper, tomatoes, mushrooms, peas, 1⅓ cup boiling water, and the thyme in a saucepan. Bring to a boil, stir well, cover, and simmer gently for about 25 minutes, until the rice is tender. Add more water during cooking if needed. Stir in the lemon rind and salt and pepper. Turn out onto a serving dish and sprinkle on the nuts.

F-Plan for People Who Work Away from Home

All the menus in this section include a brown-bag lunch, making them ideal for people who work away from home. The easiest and often the only way to stick to your diet when you have to eat lunch at work is to take your own meal with you. Those who think that brown-bag lunches must always be sandwiches will be pleasantly surprised to find that the lunches given here also include salads, soups, flatbread with toppings, pizza, and filled rolls. All are easy to pack and eat, so long as you remember to pack any necessary cutlery. Hot soups can easily be carried in a Thermos bottle; only prepared canned soups have been included, since working people do not have time to cook soup before leaving for work in the morning.

The meals for the rest of the day in each menu are breakfast (either Fiber-Filler or Bran Buds*), evening meal (usually something quick and easy, since most working people have little time for meal preparation after work), and a snack, which can be eaten anytime during the evening.

The menus are divided into two sections of approximately 1,000 and 1,250 calories. Half the menus in each section contain Fiber-Filler in the daily allowance, as in all basic F-Plan diets, and the remaining menus contain Bran Buds in the daily allowance, so that you can decide which suits you best or use both, on different days, to provide variety.

While the menus with the brown-bag lunches are just right for weekdays or workdays, you might like to have something different on the weekend. You will find plenty of choice for weekend menus in the "Simply F-Plan" (page 17) and the "Keen Cook's F-Plan" (page 103) menus.

Special Diet Notes

1. Decide on your daily calorie allowance, either 1,000 calories or 1,250 calories, which will depend on how fast you

*The analysis is based on Kellogg's Bran Buds.

want your weight loss to be, how overweight you are, and the amount of physical work you do.

2. Include as many different menus as possible from the selection provided, to keep your diet interesting and nutritious.

3. Do not swap individual meals from one menu to another, since all the menus have been carefully calculated.

4. Drink as much sugarless tea and coffee as you like, either black or with the skim milk remaining from your daily allowance after using it on the Fiber-Filler or Bran Buds. You can use artificial sweeteners. In addition, you can drink unlimited amounts of canned and bottled low-calorie-labeled drinks (Tab, Diet Pepsi, Diet Shasta, etc.), and also water and seltzer. In fact, it is often helpful to have a low-calorie fizzy drink when your willpower is flagging, since such drinks can make you feel full. Alcoholic drinks have not been included in these menus. However, there may be occasions when you feel you must have an alcoholic drink; in this case, select a 1,000-calorie menu and allow yourself drinks to the value of 200 or 250 calories from the chart on page 266.

1,000-Calorie Menu #1

	Calories	Fiber (g)
Daily allowance: Fiber-Filler, 1 cup skim milk, an orange, and an apple or pear	450	23.0
Breakfast Half portion of Fiber-Filler with milk from allowance		
Office or work lunch *Liverwurst and Cucumber Sandwich 1 small carrot stick 1 large celery stalk, cut into short sticks Apple or pear from allowance	288	5.3

Evening meal

1 chicken leg and thigh (skin removed), broiled		
½ cup canned corn		
½ cup canned mushrooms		
Orange from allowance and 10 black grapes	322	7.2

Snack

Remaining Fiber-Filler with milk from
  allowance

Total	**1,060**	**35.5**

LIVERWURST AND CUCUMBER SANDWICH Serves 1

2   large slices of whole wheat bread
1½ tablespoons Underwood Liverwurst Spread
½   medium cucumber, sliced
     Salt and pepper to taste

Spread both slices of bread with liverwurst. Top with cucumber and season with salt and pepper.

1,000-Calorie Menu #2

	Calories	Fiber (g)
Daily Allowance: Fiber-Filler, 1 cup skim milk, an orange, and an apple or pear	450	23.0

Breakfast

Half portion of Fiber-Filler with milk
  from allowance

Office or work lunch
*Ham and Fruit Salad
4 wheat crackers spread with 1 teaspoon
   diet margarine
Orange from allowance   255   5.4

Evening meal
*Cheesy Fish and Tomato Pie
⅔ cup frozen mixed peas and carrots
Apple or pear from allowance   327   8.7

Snack
Remaining Fiber-Filler with milk from
   allowance

	Total	**1,032**	**37.1**

*HAM AND FRUIT SALAD   *Serves 1*

1   (1-ounce) slice of lean boiled ham
1   small apple (in addition to allowance)
2   teaspoons lemon juice
10 black grapes, halved and seeded
2   celery stalks, chopped
1   tablespoon oil-free French dressing
   Salt and pepper to taste
   A few lettuce leaves

Trim off any fat and chop the ham. Core and chop the apple, and toss in the lemon juice to prevent browning. Mix the apple with the grapes, celery, French dressing, and salt and pepper. Arrange the lettuce leaves in the bottom of a plastic carton. Spoon the apple and grape mixture into the carton and top with the chopped ham. Remember to take a fork to work.

*CHEESY FISH AND TOMATO PIE   *Serves 1*

1   (6-ounce) package of frozen fish fillet in butter sauce
¼   cup instant mashed potatoes
1   tomato, sliced
2   tablespoons grated Parmesan cheese

Cook the fish as directed on the package. Make up instant potatoes as directed (do not add butter). Spoon the potato around the edges of the fish dish. Cover the fish with tomato slices and sprinkle on the grated cheese. Heat under the broiler until the cheese browns.

1,000-Calorie Menu #3

	Calories	Fiber (g)
Daily allowance: Fiber-Filler, 1 cup skim milk, an orange, and an apple or pear	450	23.0
Breakfast Half portion of Fiber-Filler with milk from allowance		
Office or work lunch 4 wheat crackers 1 cup coleslaw 1 (1-ounce) slice of salami (Pack the ingredients separately to keep the crackers from becoming soggy; at lunchtime, spoon the coleslaw over the crackers and top with sliced salami.) Apple or pear from allowance	228	5.7
Evening meal *Baked Potato with Sausage Topping		

⅓ cup baked beans in tomato sauce
Orange from allowance   388   10.3

Snack
Remaining Fiber-Filler with milk from
   allowance

Total	**1,066**	**39.0**

*BAKED POTATO WITH SAUSAGE TOPPING   Serves 1

1   large potato
2   Hormel brown-and-serve beef sausages
3   tablespoons corn relish

Bake the potato following one of the methods on page 20.
Grill the sausages until well done. Cut the baked potato in half
lengthwise and scoop out some of the flesh. Mix with the corn
relish and pile back into the potato jacket. Arrange a sausage
on the top of each potato half. Accompany with heated baked
beans.

1,000-Calorie Menu #4

	Calories	Fiber (g)
Daily allowance: Fiber-Filler, 1 cup skim milk, an orange, and an apple or pear	450	23.0
Breakfast Half portion of Fiber-Filler with milk from allowance ⅓ cup Bran Buds	70	8.0
Office or work lunch 1 hard-boiled egg		

Salad: a bunch of parsley, a few
   scallions, 1 celery stalk (chopped), 1
   carrot (cut into small sticks), ½
   medium cucumber (sliced), 1 tomato
   (cut into wedges), and 1 tablespoon
   oil-free French Dressing
(Put all the salad vegetables in a plastic
   container and toss in the French
   dressing. Seal the container and take
   to work, with the egg wrapped
   separately.)
4 wheat crackers (Wheat Thins), spread
   with 1 teaspoon diet margarine
Apple or pear from allowance   210   4.0

Evening meal
* Spaghetti with Tuna Sauce
4 wheat crackers (Wheat Thins), spread
   with 1 ounce Laughing Cow (triangle-
   pack) cheese
Orange from allowance   327   3.7

Snack
Remaining Fiber-Filler with milk from
   allowance

	Total	**1,057**	**38.7**

*SPAGHETTI WITH TUNA SAUCE   *Serves 1*

⅓   cup enriched spaghetti
¾   cup canned tomatoes with juice
1   tablespoon finely chopped onion
     Pinch of dried basil or oregano
½   cup water-packed tuna
     Salt and pepper to taste

Boil the spaghetti in salted water for about 12 minutes, or until
just tender. Meanwhile, purée the tomatoes with juice in a

blender, or mash well with a fork. Put in a small saucepan with the onion and herbs. Bring to a boil, cover, and simmer for 5 minutes. Flake the tuna and add to the sauce, along with salt and pepper. Stir well and continue to heat for 3 minutes. Drain the spaghetti and arrange on a serving dish. Spoon the tuna sauce over the spaghetti.

1,000-Calorie Menu #5

	Calories	Fiber (g)
Daily Allowance: Fiber-Filler, 1 cup skim milk, an orange, and an apple or pear	450	23.0
Breakfast Half portion of Fiber-Filler with milk from allowance		
Office or work lunch 1 cup canned lentil soup 4 wheat crackers (Heat soup and carry to work in a Thermos; wrap the crackers. Remember to take a spoon.) Orange from allowance	186	5.7
Evening meal *Red Onion and Herb Omelet ¾ cup fresh or frozen peas 1 cup water-packed canned peaches	376	12.5
Snack Remaining Fiber-Filler with milk from allowance Apple or pear from allowance		
Total	**1,012**	**41.2**

*RED ONION AND HERB OMELET   *Serves 1*

2   eggs
1   tablespoon water
    Salt and pepper to taste
1   tablespoon chopped fresh parsley
1   teaspoon diet margarine
½   cup chopped red onion

Beat the eggs with water, salt and pepper, and parsley. Grease a nonstick omelet pan or small frying pan with margarine and heat. Sauté onion until soft; pour in the egg mixture and cook until the bottom of the omelet is set and beginning to brown and the top is still slightly runny. Fold the omelet and turn out onto a warm plate. Accompany with peas.

1,000-Calorie Menu #6

	Calories	Fiber (g)
Daily allowance: ⅔ cup Bran Buds, 1 cup skim milk, an orange, and an apple or pear	421	24
Breakfast Half portion of Bran Buds with milk from allowance Orange from allowance		
Office or work lunch *Peanut Butter and Salad Lunch Roll 1 carrot, cut into sticks 1 large celery stalk, cut into small sticks Apple or pear from allowance	340	13

Evening meal
6 ounces frozen sole in lemon butter
⅔ cup canned corn
¾ cup cabbage, boiled
½ cup low-fat plain yogurt   268   10

Snack
Remaining Bran Buds with milk from
   allowance

Total	**1,029**	**47**

*PEANUT BUTTER AND SALAD LUNCH ROLL
Serves 1

1   whole-wheat bagel
1   tablespoon peanut butter
1   tomato, sliced
½ medium cucumber, sliced
    Chopped lettuce

Split the bagel in two and spread the bottom half with peanut butter. Top with tomato, cucumber, and lettuce. Replace the top half. Wrap.

1,000-Calorie Menu #7

	Calories	Fiber (g)
Daily allowance: ⅔ cup Bran Buds, 1 cup skim milk, an orange, and an apple or pear	421	24.0

Breakfast
Half portion of Bran Buds with milk
   from allowance
Orange from allowance

Office or work lunch
*Cottage Cheese and Grape Salad
4 wheat crackers (Wheat Thins)
1 medium banana   256   5.3

Evening meal
*Cauliflower with Chicken Liver and
   Mushroom Sauce
½ cup canned corn
Apple or pear from allowance   299   11.3

Snack
Remaining Bran Buds with milk from
   allowance

                              Total   **976**   **40.6**

*COTTAGE CHEESE AND GRAPE SALAD   *Serves 1*

½ cup cottage cheese
10 black grapes, halved and seeded
1   large celery stalk, chopped
    Salt and pepper to taste
    A few lettuce leaves, shredded

Mix cottage cheese with grapes, celery, and seasoning. Line a
plastic carton with lettuce and spoon the salad on top.

*CAULIFLOWER WITH CHICKEN LIVER AND MUSHROOM SAUCE *Serves 1*

3½ ounces chicken livers, chopped
1 tablespoon chopped onion
¼ clove garlic, crushed (optional)
1 carrot, grated
¼ chicken bouillon cube
½ cup boiling water
   Salt and pepper to taste
5 mushrooms, chopped
1½ cups cauliflower florets

Put chicken livers, onion, garlic, and carrot in a small saucepan. Dissolve the bouillon cube in ½ cup boiling water and pour into the pan. Add salt and pepper. Bring to a boil, cover, and simmer gently for 20 minutes. Add the mushrooms and simmer for 5 minutes. Meanwhile, cook the cauliflower in salted boiling water until just tender, then drain. Arrange the cauliflower on a serving dish and pour on the chicken liver and mushroom sauce.

1,000-Calorie Menu #8

	Calories	Fiber (g)
Daily allowance: ⅔ cup Bran Buds, 1 cup skim milk, an orange, and an apple or pear	421	24.0

Breakfast
Half portion of Bran Buds with milk
   from allowance
Orange from allowance

Office or work lunch
*Salmon Salad on a Roll
Apple or pear from allowance   230   2.8

Evening meal
3 (1-ounce) slices of chopped ham
    steak, grilled without fat
2 tomatoes, broiled without fat
½ cup canned baked beans with tomato
    sauce
2 tablespoons instant mashed potatoes
    made up with water (no butter)   404   16.5

Snack
Remaining Bran Buds with milk from
    allowance

Total	**1,055**	**43.3**

*SALMON SALAD ON A ROLL   *Serves 1*

1   whole-wheat roll
¼   cup flaked canned salmon
½   medium cucumber, chopped
1   teaspoon diet mayonnaise

Split the roll in half. Combine salmon, cucumber, and mayonnaise and spread on the bottom half of the roll. Top with remaining half. Wrap.

1,000-Calorie Menu #9

	Calories	**Fiber (g)**
Daily allowance: ⅔ cup Bran Buds, 1 cup skim milk, an orange, and an apple or pear	421	24.0

Breakfast
Half portion of Bran Buds with milk
   from allowance
Orange from allowance

Office or work lunch	215	8.7

1 cup Campbell's Pea and Ham Soup
4 wheat crackers (Wheat Thins)
Apple or pear from allowance

Evening meal
*Chicken with Raisin Coleslaw
   Vinaigrette
4 wheat crackers with 1 triangle of
   Laughing Cow cheese, topped with ½

cucumber, sliced	397	5.9

Snack
Remaining Bran Buds with milk from
   allowance

Total	**1,033**	**8.6**

*CHICKEN AND RAISIN COLESLAW
VINAIGRETTE*   *Serves 1*

1   chicken leg and thigh
¾   cup shredded cabbage
1   medium carrot, grated
1   large celery stalk, finely chopped
1   tablespoon raisins
1   tablespoon oil-free French dressing

Broil the chicken until cooked through. Mix the cabbage, carrot, celery, raisins, and French dressing until well blended. Remove the skin from the chicken and accompany the chicken with the coleslaw.

1,000-Calorie Menu #10

	Calories	Fiber (g)
Daily allowance: ⅔ cup Bran Buds, 1 cup skim milk, an orange, and an apple or pear	421	24.0
Breakfast Half portion of Bran Buds with milk from allowance		
Office or work lunch 2 slices of bologna 1 cup coleslaw Apple or pear from allowance	295	5.0
Evening meal *Baked Potato with Cheesy Filling ⅓ cup canned baked beans with tomato sauce Orange from allowance	315	12.3
Snack Remaining Bran Buds with milk from allowance		
Total	**1,031**	**41.3**

*BAKED POTATO WITH CHEESY FILLING   Serves 1

1	large potato
¼	cup cottage cheese with chives
1	tablespoon corn relish
	Salt and pepper to taste
2	teaspoons grated Parmesan cheese

Bake the potato following one of the methods on page 20. Cut the potato in half lengthwise and scoop out some of the flesh. Add the cottage cheese, corn relish, and salt and pepper to the potato and mash together. Pile the mixture back into the potato jacket. Sprinkle Parmesan cheese over potato halves and heat through under the broiler until the cheese begins to brown.

1,250-Calorie Menu #1

	Calories	Fiber (g)
Daily allowance: Fiber-Filler, 1 cup skim milk, an orange, and an apple or pear	450	23.0
Breakfast Half portion of Fiber-Filler with milk from allowance Orange from allowance		
Office or work lunch *Deviled Egg Sandwich ½ cup plain low-fat yogurt Apple or pear from allowance	353	6.2
Evening meal *Thatched Cod and Broccoli ½ cup fresh or frozen green beans 25 green grapes	418	11.0
Snack Remaining Fiber-Filler with milk from allowance 2 whole-wheat crackers spread with 2 tablespoons cottage cheese with chives	52	0.9
Total	**1,273**	**41.1**

*DEVILED EGG SANDWICH   *Serves 1*

1   tablespoon diet mayonnaise
¼   teaspoon Worcestershire sauce
1   medium carrot, grated
2   large slices of Pepperidge Farm whole-wheat bread
1   hard-boiled egg, sliced
2   lettuce leaves, chopped

Mix the mayonnaise with Worcestershire sauce and carrot. Divide between the slices of bread. Arrange the egg slices and lettuce on one slice of bread and cover with the second slice.

*THATCHED COD AND BROCCOLI   *Serves 1*

1⅓ cups frozen broccoli
4   ounces frozen sole in lemon butter sauce
     Salt and pepper to taste
2   tablespoons fresh whole-wheat bread crumbs
1   tablespoon grated Cheddar cheese

Cook the broccoli and sole according to package directions. Drain the broccoli and season with salt and pepper. Put in a shallow ovenproof dish. Put the sole and sauce on the broccoli. Mix the bread crumbs with grated cheese and sprinkle on top. Heat under the broiler until topping is crisp and golden brown.

1,250-Calorie Menu #2

	Calories	Fiber (g)
Daily allowance: Fiber-Filler, 1 cup skim milk, an orange, and an apple or pear	450	23.0
Breakfast		
Half portion of Fiber-Filler with milk from allowance		
1 large slice of whole-wheat bread, toasted and spread with 1 teaspoon diet margarine and 1 teaspoon marmalade or honey	100	1.3
Office or work lunch		
1 regular McDonald's hamburger on a bun		
Orange from allowance	257	0.8
Evening meal		
1 pork chop, broiled and with fat cut off; with 1 slice of juice-packed pineapple, heated under the broiler		
¾ cup canned button mushrooms, heated through and drained		
¾ cup frozen peas, boiled		
½ cup vanilla ice cream		
Apple or pear from allowance	498	13.6
Snack		
Remaining Fiber-Filler with milk from allowance		
Total	**1,305**	**38.7**

1,250-Calorie Menu #3

	Calories	Fiber (g)
Daily allowance: Fiber-Filler, 1 cup skim milk, an orange, and an apple or pear	450	23.0
Breakfast Half portion of Fiber-Filler with milk from allowance 1 medium banana	85	2.7
Office or work lunch *Corned Beef and Corn Relish Lunch Roll 1 large carrot, sliced Orange from allowance	294	7.3
Evening meal *Grilled Spiced Chicken with Stir-Fry Vegetables Apple or pear from allowance	502	7.0
Snack Remaining Fiber-Filler with milk from allowance		
Total	**1,331**	**40.0**

*CORNED BEEF AND CORN RELISH LUNCH
ROLL   *Serves 1*

1   whole-wheat lunch roll
1   teaspoon mustard

2   (1-ounce) slices of corned beef
2   tablespoons corn relish
2   lettuce leaves, chopped

Split the roll in two and spread with mustard. Arrange the corned beef on the bottom half of the roll and top with relish and lettuce. Top with other half of the roll.

*GRILLED SPICED CHICKEN WITH STIR-FRY VEGETABLES *Serves 1*

1   chicken leg and thigh
2   tablespoons Saucy Susan spicy sauce
1½ cups Birds Eye Stir-Fry Vegetables

Remove the skin from the chicken and brush all over with sauce. Broil until cooked through. Meanwhile, cook the vegetables according to the package directions. Accompany chicken with vegetables.

1,250-Calorie Menu #4

	Calories	Fiber (g)
Daily allowance: Fiber-Filler, 1 cup skim milk, an orange, and an apple or pear	450	23.0

Breakfast
Half portion of Fiber-Filler with milk
  from allowance
Orange from allowance

1 egg, poached and served on 1 large slice of Arnold whole-wheat bread, toasted and spread with 1 tablespoon tomato ketchup	153	1.2

Office or work lunch
1 cup Progresso Lentil Soup
4 wheat crackers

Apple or pear from allowance	186	5.7

Evening meal
1 (3½-ounce) loin lamb chop, broiled
12 Brussels sprouts, boiled
⅔ cup carrots, boiled

1 large slice of juice-packed pineapple	451	7.3

Snack
Remaining Fiber-Filler with milk from
allowance

1 medium carrot, cut into sticks	21	1.6
Total	**1,261**	**38.8**

1,250-Calorie Menu #5

	Calories	Fiber (g)
Daily allowance: Fiber-Filler, 1 cup skim milk, an orange, and an apple or pear	450	23.0

Breakfast
Half portion of Fiber-Filler with milk
from allowance

1 large slice of whole-wheat bread, toasted and spread with 1 teaspoon diet margarine and 1 teaspoon marmalade or honey	100	1.4

Office or work lunch
2 (1-ounce) slices of lean boiled ham
   with any fat trimmed off
4 wheat crackers spread with 1 teaspoon
   diet margarine
¾ cup coleslaw
Apple or pear from allowance   273   4.5

Evening meal
*Baked Potato with Egg and Tomato
   Filling
⅓ cup canned baked beans with tomato
   sauce
¼ cup vanilla ice cream
Orange from allowance   437   13.6

Snack
Remaining Fiber-Filler with milk from
   allowance
½ medium banana   45   1.4
                                         _____
                        Total   **1,305**   **43.9**

*BAKED POTATO WITH EGG AND TOMATO
FILLING   *Serves 1*

1   large potato
1   egg
2   tablespoons skim milk from allowance
1   teaspoon margarine
    Salt and pepper to taste
1   medium tomato, chopped

Bake the potato according to the directions on page 20. Scramble the egg with the skim milk, margarine, and salt and pepper in a small saucepan. Stir in the tomato and heat through. Cut the potato in half lengthwise and scoop out some of the flesh. Mash the potato flesh and mix with the scrambled egg and tomato. Pile back into the potato jacket.

1,250-Calorie Menu #6

	Calories	Fiber (g)
This menu is suitable for vegetarians.		
Daily allowance: ⅔ cup Bran Buds, 1 cup skim milk, an orange, and an apple or pear	421	24.0
Breakfast Half portion of Bran Buds with milk from allowance Orange from allowance		
Office or work lunch *Waldorf Salad 1 Nature Valley granola bar	389	8.2
Evening meal *One-Pan Pasta Dish Apple or pear from allowance	407	5.8
Snack Remaining Bran Buds with milk from allowance		
Total	**1,217**	**38.0**

*WALDORF SALAD   *Serves 1*

1   cup shredded cabbage
1   large celery stalk, chopped
1   small apple (in addition to allowance), cored and
    chopped
2   teaspoons lemon juice
1   tablespoon chopped walnuts
2   tablespoons diet mayonnaise

Mix together the cabbage and celery. Toss the apple in the lemon juice and then add to the cabbage and celery, along with the walnuts and mayonnaise. Mix well.

*ONE-PAN PASTA DISH   *Serves 1*

⅔   cup whole-wheat spaghetti or macaroni
1   teaspoon diet margarine
1   small onion, peeled and chopped
5   mushrooms, sliced
1   medium tomato, chopped
2   eggs
4   tablespoons skim milk (in addition to allowance)
    Salt and pepper to taste
1   tablespoon grated Cheddar cheese

Boil the spaghetti in salted water for about 12 minutes, or until just tender. Heat the margarine in a pan, add the onion, and cook gently until soft. Add the mushrooms and tomato and cook for 3 to 4 minutes. Add the drained spaghetti and heat through. Beat the eggs with milk and salt and pepper. Pour over the pasta mixture and cook over a low heat, stirring continuously, until sauce begins to thicken. Do not allow to boil. Remove from heat and sprinkle with grated cheese.

1,250-Calorie Menu #7

	Calories	Fiber (g)

This menu is suitable for vegetarians.

Daily allowance: ⅔ cup Bran Buds, 1
   cup skim milk, an orange, and an
   apple or pear | 421 | 24.0

Breakfast
Half portion of Bran Buds with milk
   from allowance
2 whole-wheat crackers spread with 1
   teaspoon honey | 52 | 0.9

Office or work lunch
1 envelope of Lipton's Cup-of-Soup
   (noodle)
Cheese, tomato, and cucumber
   sandwich: 2 large slices of Arnold
   whole-wheat bread spread with 1
   triangle of Laughing Cow cheese,
   topped with 1 medium tomato (sliced)
   and a few slices of cucumber
Apple or pear from allowance | 281 | 4.6

Evening meal
* Vegetable and Cheese Pie
4 wheat crackers (Wheat Thins)
Orange from allowance | 469 | 23.4

Snack
Remaining Bran Buds with milk from
   allowance
½ cup low-fat plain yogurt | 45 |

| **Total** | **1,268** | **52.9** |

*VEGETABLE AND CHEESE PIE *Serves 1*

2 teaspoons diet margarine
1 tablespoon whole-wheat flour
½ cup skim milk (in addition to allowance)
    Salt and pepper to taste
¼ teaspoon mustard
2 tablespoons grated Cheddar cheese
¾ cup canned lima beans
⅔ cup frozen mixed vegetables

Put margarine, flour, and milk in a small saucepan and heat gently, stirring constantly, until the mixture boils and thickens. Season with salt and pepper and stir in the mustard and half the grated cheese. Remove from the heat. Heat the can of lima beans and drain. Cook the mixed vegetables according to package directions and drain. Mix the beans and mixed vegetables with the cheese sauce and turn into a small ovenproof dish. Sprinkle on the remaining cheese and heat under the broiler until the cheese is melted and beginning to brown.

1,250-Calorie Menu #8

	Calories	Fiber (g)
Daily allowance: ⅔ cup Bran Buds, 1 cup skim milk, an orange, and an apple or pear	421	24.0

Breakfast
Half portion of Bran Buds with milk
   from allowance

Office or work lunch
1 slice of Pizza Hut pizza
Mixed salad: a few lettuce leaves
   (shredded), 1 tomato (cut into
   wedges), a few cucumber slices, a
   few scallions (chopped)
Apple or pear from allowance   220   4.1

Evening meal
*Bean and Frankfurter Supper
¼ cup vanilla ice cream
Orange from allowance   524   25.9

Snack
Half portion of Bran Buds with milk
   from allowance
1 large slice of Arnold whole-wheat
   bread toasted and spread with 1
   triangle Laughing Cow cheese   139   1.2

	Total	**1,304**	**55.2**

*BEAN AND FRANKFURTER SUPPER   Serves 1

¾   cup canned baked beans with tomato sauce
1   teaspoon Worcestershire sauce
¼   teaspoon mustard
1   tablespoon finely chopped onion
1   tomato, chopped
2   tablespoons tomato juice
1   frankfurter, sliced and cooked
1   large slice of Arnold whole-wheat bread

Mix together all the ingredients except the bread in a saucepan. Heat to a simmer, cover, and cook over low heat for 15
minutes. Meanwhile, toast the bread. Pile the bean and frankfurter mixture on the toast.

1,250-Calorie Menu #9

	Calories	Fiber (g)
Daily allowance: ⅔ cup Bran Buds, 1 cup skim milk, an orange, and an apple or pear	421	24.0
Breakfast Half portion of Bran Buds with milk from allowance 1 egg, poached and served on 1 large slice of whole-wheat bread, toasted and spread with 1 teaspoon diet margarine	159	2.1
Office or work lunch Cottage cheese and date sandwich: 2 large slices of whole-wheat bread filled with ⅓ cup cottage cheese mixed with 2 tablespoons chopped dates Apple or pear from allowance	293	5.8
Evening meal *Tuna and Corn in Sauce with Cauliflower ½ cup juice-packed peach slices 2 tablespoons plain low-fat yogurt	362	8.5
Snack Remaining Bran Buds with milk from allowance Orange from allowance		
Total	**1,235**	**40.4**

TUNA AND CORN IN SAUCE WITH CAULIFLOWER   *Serves 1*

½   chicken bouillon cube
½   cup skim milk (in addition to allowance)
1   tablespoon whole-wheat flour
½   cup water-packed tuna, drained and flaked
⅓   cup canned corn
1   cup cauliflower florets

Dissolve bouillon cube in milk; add flour and blend well. Bring slowly to boil, stirring continuously. Lower the heat, continue to stir, and simmer for 3 minutes. Add the tuna and corn and heat through. Cook the cauliflower in boiling water until just tender, about 10 minutes. Drain well and arrange on a serving dish. Pour the sauce over the cauliflower.

1,250-Calorie Menu #10

	Calories	Fiber (g)
Daily allowance: ⅔ cup Bran Buds, 1 cup skim milk, an orange, and an apple or pear	421	24.0
Breakfast Full portion of Bran Buds with milk from allowance Apple or pear from allowance		
Office or work lunch *Kidney Bean, Mushroom, Corn, and Cheese Salad Orange from allowance	300	14.0
Evening meal *Liver and Bacon in a Pot ¼ cup instant mashed potatoes made up with boiling water (no butter)	377	7.2

Snack
1 large slice of whole-wheat bread,
    toasted, topped with ¼ cup grated
    mozzarella cheese, heated under the
    broiler until the cheese melts   144   1.2

Total	**1,242**	**46.4**

*KIDNEY BEAN, MUSHROOM, CORN, AND CHEESE SALAD *Serves 1*

⅓   cup canned kidney beans, drained
5   mushrooms, sliced
⅓   cup canned corn
¼   cup diced Swiss cheese
2   tablespoons oil-free French dressing

Mix all the ingredients well. Pack in a plastic carton.

*LIVER AND BACON IN A POT *Serves 1*

1   teaspoon diet margarine
1   slice of Canadian bacon, chopped
1   medium carrot, sliced
1   small onion, peeled and sliced
3½ ounces chicken livers, thinly sliced
¾   cup canned tomatoes
    Pinch of dried thyme
    Salt and pepper to taste

Melt the margarine in a saucepan and add the bacon, carrot, and onion. Cover and cook gently for 5 minutes, shaking the pan from time to time. Turn into a small ovenproof casserole and lay the liver slices on top. Chop the tomatoes in their juice and spoon over the liver. Sprinkle on the thyme and season well with salt and pepper. Cover and cook in a slow oven at 300°F for 1 hour. Serve with mashed potato.

Snack Eater's F-Plan

Some people tend to eat frequent snacks. If this pattern of eating is your norm, these menus of five small snack meals a day will provide your easiest F-Plan method. And there is no harm—you may even lose weight slightly faster—in eating little and often, so long as your total food and fiber intake is correct for the day.

The menus all follow the basic F-Plan rules (page 12). The snack meals are all simple and quick to prepare, both to reduce to a minimum the time spent in the kitchen and because snack eaters and nibblers tend to prefer more or less instant foods.

As with the "Simply F-Plan" menus, these snack eater's menus are divided into two sections—menus providing approximately 1,000 calories and menus providing 1,250 calories daily—to enable you to choose menus that will result in the best weight loss for you.

Special Diet Rules

1. Decide which daily calorie total will give you the best weight loss. For guidance on the most suitable daily calorie allowance for you, see page 15.

2. Plan ahead and select at least two or three menus (preferably one week's menus) at a time, to enable you to shop for the foods you need.

3. Make sure that you eat a variety of foods by selecting several different menus each week, to be sure that you are getting all the nutrients you need for good health.

4. The five snack meals from your daily menu can be eaten in any order and at any time of day you wish. However, it is inadvisable to swap one snack meal from one menu with a meal from another menu, since this will usually alter the amount of calories and fiber that has been carefully counted for each full day's menu.

5. Drinks can be taken at any time during the day and in any quantity, provided that you stick to sugarless tea and coffee, either black or with skim milk from the daily allowance (reserve some to eat with the Fiber-Filler), low-calorie-labeled bottled and canned drinks, and water. If you feel the need to have an alcoholic drink occasionally, see the advice given on page 266 and select a drink from the chart.

1,000-Calorie Menu #1

	Calories	Fiber (g)
Daily allowance: Fiber-Filler, 1 cup skim milk, an orange, and an apple or pear	450	23.0
Meal 1 Half portion of Fiber-Filler with milk from allowance		
Meal 2 1 egg, poached and served on 1 large slice of Arnold whole-wheat bread, toasted and spread with 1 teaspoon diet margarine	159	1.2
Meal 3 1 cup Progresso Lentil Soup 2 whole-wheat crackers 2 tablespoons cottage cheese and chives Apple or pear from allowance	182	5.8
Meal 4 2 frozen fish cakes (4 ounces), baked 1 medium tomato, halved and broiled ¾ cup frozen peas	258	8.7

Meal 5
Remaining Fiber-Filler with
milk from allowance
Orange from allowance

	Total	1,049	38.7

1,000-Calorie Menu #2

	Calories	Fiber (g)
Daily allowance: Fiber-Filler, 1 cup skim milk, an orange, and an apple or pear	450	23.0

Meal 1
Half portion of Fiber-Filler with milk
   from allowance
Orange from allowance

Meal 2

Cottage cheese and cucumber sandwich: 2 large slices of Pepperidge Farm whole-wheat bread filled with ¼ cup cottage cheese (plain, with chives, with onions and peppers, or with pineapple), salt and pepper to taste, and ½ medium cucumber (sliced)	158	3.1

Meal 3

½ cup low-fat yogurt, mixed with 1 sliced medium banana and 2 chopped walnut halves	154	2.9

Meal 4

1 (4 ounces raw) hamburger, broiled 1 medium tomato, broiled ½ cup baked beans in tomato sauce	312	14.0

Meal 5
Remaining Fiber-Filler with milk from
   allowance
Apple or pear from allowance

	Total	1,074	43.0

1,000-Calorie Menu #3

	Calories	Fiber (g)
Daily allowance: Fiber-Filler, 1 cup skim milk, an orange, and an apple or pear	450	23.0

Meal 1
Half portion of Fiber-Filler with milk
   from allowance
Orange from allowance

Meal 2
3 whole-wheat crackers, each topped
   with tomato slices
1 sardine canned in tomato sauce
1 chopped sour pickle
Apple from allowance   210   4.4

Meal 3
4 canned prunes with 2 tablespoons
   juice
1 tablespoon low-fat yogurt   185   8.1

Meal 4
4 ounces cod steak, covered with 1
   tablespoon chopped onion, ½ cup
   canned tomatoes, salt and pepper to
   taste, and a pinch of mixed herbs,
   covered and baked at 350°F for 25
   minutes
⅔ cup frozen mixed vegetables, boiled   159   7.7

Meal 5
Remaining Fiber-Filler with milk from
 allowance
2 whole-wheat crackers spread with 1
 teaspoon margarine and topped with
 ⅓ cup grated carrot

	Calories	Fiber (g)
(Meal 5)	62	1.9
Total	**1,066**	**45.1**

1,000-Calorie Menu #4

	Calories	Fiber (g)
Daily allowance: Fiber-Filler, 1 cup skim milk, an orange, and an apple or pear	450	23.0

Meal 1
Half portion of Fiber-Filler with milk
 from allowance
2 whole-wheat crackers, topped with 1
 piece of gefilte fish spread with 1
 teaspoon horseradish — 82, 0.9

Meal 2
2 slices of bacon, broiled, with ⅓ cup
 baked beans in tomato sauce and 1
 tomato, halved — 263, 9.5

Meal 3
½ cup cottage cheese (plain or with
 pineapple)
Salad: a few lettuce leaves, ½ cucumber
 (sliced), 1 medium tomato (sliced), 2
 scallions (chopped), 1 ring of red
 pepper (chopped), 1 celery stalk

(chopped), and 1 tablespoon oil-free
French dressing
2 whole-wheat crackers   138   4.0

Meal 4
1 small ½-ounce package of Lay's
    potato chips
2 large celery stalks
½ cup low-fat yogurt   128   1.5

Meal 5
Remaining Fiber-Filler with milk from
    allowance
Orange and apple or pear from
    allowance

	Total	**1,061**	**38.9**

1,000-Calorie Menu #5

	Calories	**Fiber (g)**

Daily allowance: Fiber-Filler, 1 cup
    skim milk, an orange, and an apple or
    pear   450   23.0

Meal 1
Half portion of Fiber-Filler with milk
    from allowance
Orange from allowance

Meal 2
Ham and pickle sandwich: 2 large slices
    of Pepperidge Farm whole-wheat
    bread spread with 1 tablespoon sweet
    pickle relish, with 1 (1-ounce) slice of
    ham and ½ medium cucumber (sliced)
Apple or pear from allowance   234   4.5

Meal 3
Mexican omelet: Beat 2 eggs with 2
   tablespoons water and salt and
   pepper. Grease a small nonstick
   omelet pan with a little diet
   margarine. Heat the pan, add the egg
   mixture, and cook until the egg is just
   set. Spoon ½ cup canned corn with 1
   tablespoon chopped green pepper into
   the center. Fold the omelet in half and
   serve with chopped lettuce.   261   4.6

Meal 4
½ cup juice-packed pear halves
1 tablespoon low-fat yogurt   70   3.9

Meal 5
Remaining Fiber-Filler with milk from
   allowance
1 large celery stalk with 2 tablespoons
   cottage cheese   23   1.0

	Total	1,038	37.0

1,000-Calorie Menu #6

	Calories	Fiber (g)
Daily allowance: Fiber-Filler, 1 cup skim milk, an orange, and an apple or pear	450	23.0
Meal 1		
Half portion of Fiber-Filler with milk from allowance		
1 medium banana	85	2.7

Meal 2

1 envelope Lipton's Cup-a-Soup (noodle)		
4 whole-wheat crackers, each spread with 1 tablespoon low-fat cottage cheese and topped with 2½ tablespoons grated carrot	192	3.4

Meal 3

½ cup yogurt mixed with 2 tablespoons bran		
Orange from allowance	63	2.2

Meal 4

4 ounces frozen sole in lemon butter		
¾ cup frozen peas	288	7.2

Meal 5

Remaining Fiber-Filler with milk from allowance		
Apple or pear from allowance		
Total	**1,078**	**38.5**

1,000-Calorie Menu #7

	Calories	Fiber (g)
Daily allowance: Fiber-Filler, 1 cup skim milk, an orange, and an apple or pear	450	23.0
Meal 1		
Half portion of Fiber-Filler with ½ cup plain low-fat yogurt	45	0.0

Meal 2

1 egg, boiled, with 1 large slice of Arnold whole-wheat bread spread with 1 teaspoon diet margarine		
Orange from allowance	149	1.2

Meal 3

½ cup cottage cheese, mixed with apple or pear from allowance (cored and chopped) and 2 tablespoons raisins, served on a bed of lettuce leaves and garnished with ⅔ cup grated carrot	180	4.4

Meal 4

Bean and tomato hot pot: Heat ½ cup canned beans in tomato sauce with ½ cup canned tomatoes, a generous dash of Worcestershire sauce, and pepper to taste. Broil 1 slice of Canadian bacon until crisp. Pour the bean and tomato mixture into a soup bowl and crumble the bacon over the top.	236	14.0

Meal 5

Remaining Fiber-Filler with milk from
allowance

Total	**1,060**	**42.6**

1,000-Calorie Menu #8

	Calories	Fiber (g)
Daily allowance: Fiber-Filler, 1 cup skim milk, an orange, and an apple or pear	450	23.0

Meal 1

Half portion of Fiber-Filler with milk
from allowance

Meal 2
1 Fibermed™ * biscuit
1 medium banana   145   7.7

Meal 3
½ cup canned chili con carne
¾ cup cabbage, boiled
Orange from allowance   215   8.4

Meal 4
1 cup Progresso Lentil Soup
Apple or pear from allowance   150   5.0

Meal 5
Remaining Fiber-Filler with milk from
   allowance
2 whole-wheat crackers
1 sliced piece of gefilte fish with 1
   teaspoon horseradish   82   0.9

	Total	**1,042**	**45.0**

1,000-Calorie Menu #9

	Calories	Fiber (g)

Daily allowance: Fiber-Filler, 1 cup
   skim milk, an orange, and an apple or
   pear   450   23.0

Meal 1
Half portion of Fiber-Filler with milk
   from allowance
Orange from allowance

*Available from the Purdue Frederick Co., Norwalk, CT 06856.

Meal 2

¾ cup canned baked beans in tomato
   sauce served on 1 large slice of
   Arnold whole-wheat bread, toasted   280   24.2

Meal 3

¾ cup cooked shrimp, served with a few
   lettuce leaves, ½ cucumber (sliced), 1
   medium tomato (sliced), 1 large
   celery stalk, 1 ring of green pepper,
   and 1 tablespoon oil-free French
   dressing

Apple or pear from allowance   137   4.6

Meal 4

5 water-packed apricot halves
¼ cup vanilla ice cream
2 tablespoons toasted bran
(Top the canned apricots with the ice
   cream and sprinkle with the toasted
   bran.)   148   4.7

Meal 5

Remaining Fiber-Filler with milk from
   allowance
½ cup plain low-fat yogurt   45   0.0

	Total	**1,060**	**56.5**

1,000-Calorie Menu #10

	Calories	Fiber (g)
Daily allowance: Fiber-Filler, 1 cup skim milk, an orange, and an apple or pear	450	23.0

Meal 1
Half portion of Fiber-Filler with milk
   from allowance

Meal 2
1 large slice of Arnold whole-wheat
   bread, toasted, topped with 1 sliced
   tomato, sprinkled with a pinch of
   dried thyme and salt and pepper, and
   covered with ¼ cup grated Cheddar
   cheese. Broil until the cheese is
   melted and beginning to brown.
Apple or pear from allowance   191   2.7

Meal 3
1 cup coleslaw
1 (1-ounce) slice of lean boiled ham
2 tablespoons pickled beets
2 whole-wheat crackers   232   6.1

Meal 4
¼ cup vanilla ice cream
Orange from allowance
1 Fiber-Med biscuit   132   5.0

Meal 5
Remaining Fiber-Filler with milk from
   allowance
2 whole-wheat crackers
1 tablespoon pickle relish   53   1.2
                                          ─────────────────
                          Total   **1,058**   **38.0**

1,250-Calorie Menu #1

	Calories	Fiber (g)
Daily allowance: Fiber-Filler, 1 cup skim milk, an orange, and an apple or pear	450	23.0
Meal 1 Half portion of Fiber-Filler with milk from allowance 1 large slice of Pepperidge Farm whole-wheat bread with 1 teaspoon diet margarine and 1 teaspoon honey or marmalade	113	1.5
Meal 2 2 frozen fish sticks (1 ounce each), baked ½ cup canned tomatoes, heated ¾ cup canned button mushrooms, heated and drained	160	7.0
Meal 3 ½ cup low-fat yogurt with apple or pear from allowance, cored and chopped 2 tablespoons raisins	103	1.4
Meal 4 1 cup packaged macaroni and cheese ¾ cup frozen peas, boiled ¾ cup carrots, boiled Orange from allowance	350	10.7
Meal 5 Remaining Fiber-Filler with milk from allowance 1 Fibermed biscuit spread with 1 tablespoon Underwood deviled ham	107	5.0
Total	**1,283**	**48.6**

1,250-Calorie Menu #2

	Calories	Fiber (g)
Daily allowance: Fiber-Filler, 1 cup skim milk, an orange, and an apple or pear	450	23.0
Meal 1 Half portion of Fiber-Filler with milk from allowance 1 medium banana	85	2.7
Meal 2 2 large slices of Pepperidge Farm whole-wheat bread, toasted and spread with ¼ cup cottage cheese mixed with 2 tablespoons corn relish, topped with 2 medium tomatoes (sliced), heated under the broiler Apple or pear from allowance	258	6.4
Meal 3 Remaining Fiber-Filler with milk from allowance Orange from allowance		
Meal 4 4 ounces calf's liver, sliced, brushed with 1 teaspoon oil 1 slice of bacon, broiled 1 medium tomato, halved and broiled ¾ cup cabbage, cooked	273	4.7
Meal 5 1 cup Progresso Lentil Soup 2 whole-wheat crackers	182	5.8
Total	**1,248**	**42.6**

1,250-Calorie Menu #3

	Calories	Fiber (g)
Daily allowance: Fiber-Filler, 1 cup skim milk, an orange, and an apple or pear	450	23.0
Meal 1		
Half portion of Fiber-Filler with milk from allowance		
4 whole-wheat crackers, with 1 teaspoon diet margarine and 2 teaspoons honey or marmalade	117	2.0
Meal 2		
Banana, honey, and raisin sandwich: 2 large slices of Arnold whole-wheat bread, filled with banana mashed with 2 teaspoons honey and mixed with 2 tablespoons raisins		
Apple or pear from allowance	339	6.5
Meal 3		
1 cup plain low-fat yogurt		
¼ cup bran		
1 peach	165	6.8
Meal 4		
½ cup canned Spaghetti O's topped with 1 teaspoon Parmesan cheese	168	2.3
Meal 5		
Remaining Fiber-Filler with milk from allowance		
Orange from allowance		
Total	**1,239**	**40.6**

1,250-Calorie Menu #4

	Calories	Fiber (g)
Daily allowance: Fiber-Filler, 1 cup skim milk, an orange, and an apple or pear	450	23.0
Meal 1 Half portion of Fiber-Filler with milk from allowance Orange from allowance		
Meal 2 1 Fibermed Apple/Currant biscuit ½ cup plain low-fat yogurt	105	5.0
Meal 3 1 (3-ounce) hamburger, broiled, served on a whole-wheat English muffin, with 1 tablespoon chopped sweet pickle; serve with 2 or 3 chopped lettuce leaves and 1 medium tomato	335	4.9
Meal 4 Remaining Fiber-Filler with milk from allowance 2 wheat crackers (Wheat Thins), each spread with 1 tablespoon low-fat cottage cheese with chives and 1 sliced medium tomato	74	2.4
Meal 5 1 chicken leg and thigh, broiled and skin removed ¾ cup canned corn 12 Brussels sprouts, boiled Apple or pear from allowance	369	8.5
Total	**1,333**	**43.8**

1,250-Calorie Menu #5

	Calories	Fiber (g)
Daily allowance: Fiber-Filler, 1 cup skim milk, an orange, and an apple or pear	450	23.0
Meal 1 Half portion of Fiber-Filler with milk from allowance 1 large slice of Pepperidge Farm whole-wheat bread, toasted, spread with 1 teaspoon diet margarine and 1 teaspoon honey or marmalade	113	1.2
Meal 2 ½ cup cottage cheese with pineapple coleslaw: ¾ cup finely shredded white cabbage mixed with ⅔ cup grated carrot, 1 tablespoon raisins, and 1 tablespoon diet mayonnaise	212	4.6
Meal 3 1 large slice of juice-packed pineapple ¼ cup vanilla ice cream 2 tablespoons toasted bran (Serve pineapple with ice cream, topped with bran.)	149	3.2
Meal 4 2 Jones brown-and-serve dinner sausages, broiled ½ cup baked beans in tomato sauce Orange from allowance	330	12.5

Meal 5
Remaining Fiber-Filler with milk from
    allowance
Apple or pear from allowance

	Total	1,254	44.5

1,250-Calorie Menu #6

	Calories	Fiber (g)
Daily allowance: Fiber-Filler, 1 cup skim milk, an orange, and an apple or pear	450	23.0
Meal 1 Half portion of Fiber-Filler with milk from allowance ½ toasted whole-wheat English muffin with 1 teaspoon peanut butter	97	1.7
Meal 2 1 hard-boiled egg, halved, with ½ cup three-bean salad, 2 or 3 chopped lettuce leaves, and 1 sliced tomato 2 whole-wheat crackers	278	19.1
Meal 3 1 Nature Valley Honey n' Oats Granola Bar Orange from allowance	150	1.0
Meal 4 1 (1-ounce) slice of Canadian bacon, broiled, served with 1 juice-packed pineapple ring ½ cup canned corn kernels 12 Brussels sprouts, boiled	253	7.8

Meal 5

Remaining Fiber-Filler with milk from
  allowance
2 whole-wheat crackers spread with 1
  teaspoon diet margarine, topped with
  a few cucumber slices   56   1.6
Apple or pear from allowance

	Total	**1,284**	**54.2**

1,250-Calorie Menu #7

	Calories	**Fiber (g)**

Daily allowance: Fiber-Filler, 1 cup
  skim milk, an orange, and an apple or
  pear   450   23.0

Meal 1

Half portion of Fiber-Filler with milk
  from allowance
1 medium banana   85   2.7

Meal 2

Sardines and tomato on toast: 2 large
  slices of Pepperidge Farm whole-
  wheat bread, toasted, each slice
  topped with 1 sliced medium tomato,
  a pinch of dried thyme, and 1½
  sardines in tomato sauce, heated
  under the broiler   349   3.9

Meal 3

½ cup cottage cheese with chives
1 large celery stalk, cut into small sticks
1 large carrot, cut into sticks
Apple or pear from allowance   127   3.5

Meal 4

	Calories	Fiber (g)
1 package of Green Giant boil-in-bag Gravy and Lean Roast Chicken		
¾ cup frozen peas, boiled		
2 tablespoons canned mushrooms (heat with peas)	294	8.0

Meal 5

Remaining Fiber-Filler with milk from allowance

Orange from allowance

Total	**1,305**	**41.1**

1,250-Calorie Menu #8

	Calories	Fiber (g)
Daily allowance: Fiber-Filler, 1 cup skim milk, an orange, and an apple or pear	450	23.0

Meal 1

	Calories	Fiber (g)
Half portion of Fiber-Filler with milk from allowance		
4 whole-wheat crackers spread with 1 teaspoon diet margarine and 2 teaspoons honey	120	1.6

Meal 2

	Calories	Fiber (g)
2 tablespoons Underwood Chicken Spread		
Apple or pear from allowance (cut into wedges and spread with the chicken spread)		
½ cup canned corn drizzled with oil-free salad dressing	204	3.6

Meal 3

1 package of Cup-of-Noodles		
Orange from allowance	200	0.0

Meal 4

Egg Florentine: Thaw and heat ¾ cup frozen chopped spinach (don't add butter); season to taste with salt and pepper and grated nutmeg. Put in a small ovenproof dish. Top with 1 poached egg, cover with 3 tablespoons yogurt, and sprinkle on ¼ cup grated Swiss cheese; heat under broiler until cheese begins to melt.	236	9.5

Meal 5

Remaining Fiber-Filler with milk from allowance		
1 medium banana	85	2.7
Total	**1,295**	**40.4**

1,250-Calorie Menu #9

	Calories	Fiber (g)
Daily allowance: Fiber-Filler, 1 cup skim milk, an orange, and an apple or pear	450	23.0

Meal 1

Half portion of Fiber-Filler with milk from allowance		
½ cup plain low-fat yogurt	45	0.0

Meal 2
1 cup canned macaroni and cheese
2 medium tomatoes, sliced
Apple or pear from allowance   271   3.0

Meal 3
1 Nature Valley granola bar
½ medium banana   193   3.8

Meal 4
2 Morning Star Farm frozen sausages
½ cup canned baked beans in tomato
   sauce
Orange from allowance   350   13.5

Meal 5
Remaining Fiber-Filled with milk from
   allowance
2 whole-wheat crackers
1 large celery stalk   35   1.2

	Total	**1,344**	**44.5**

1,250-Calorie Menu #10

	Calories	Fiber (g)

Daily allowance: Fiber-Filler, 1 cup
   skim milk, an orange, and an apple or
   pear   450   23.0

Meal 1
Half portion of Fiber-Filler with milk
   from allowance
1 large slice of Pepperidge Farm whole-
   wheat bread, toasted, spread with 1
   teaspoon diet margarine and 1
   teaspoon honey or marmalade   114   1.2

Meal 2
Cottage cheese and date sandwich: 2
 large slices of Pepperidge Farm
 whole-wheat bread filled with ¼ cup
 cottage cheese mixed with 2
 tablespoons chopped dates
Orange from allowance   225   4.1

Meal 3
1½ cups juice-packed peach slices
2 tablespoons low-fat yogurt   89   3.8

Meal 4
Mushroom omelet with vegetables: Beat
 2 eggs with 2 tablespoons water, salt
 and pepper to taste, and a pinch of
 dried basil. Grease a small nonstick
 omelet pan with 1 teaspoon diet
 margarine. Pour in the egg mixture
 and cook until just set. Spoon ¾ cup
 canned sliced large mushrooms
 (drained) over half the omelet. Fold
 the other half over the mushrooms
 and turn out onto a warmed plate,
 accompanied by ⅔ cup mixed
 vegetables.
Apple or pear from allowance   266   11.4

Meal 5
Remaining Fiber-Filler with milk from
 allowance   125   0.0
Chocolate drink: 1 teaspoon chocolate
 syrup and ¾ cup skim milk (in
 addition to allowance)

                                        Total   **1,269**   **43.5**

Keen Cook's F-Plan

F-Plan dieters who are also good cooks may wish to spend more time preparing their food than the majority of dieters. If you are a keen cook (male or female) and can resist the temptation to nibble while in the kitchen, you will find plenty of choice of attractive, tasty dishes to prepare in these menus.

All the recipes are for two, since if you are going to take time preparing a dish it is more worthwhile if you are sharing it with at least one other person. The ingredients can be increased proportionally if you are feeding more than two people.

Since good cooks usually prefer to spend most of their time preparing one main meal, these menus provide simple, light meals during the day, saving most of the calorie allowance for the main evening meal. A late-afternoon snack has been included in each menu to help you avoid hunger pangs and to reduce the temptation to nibble while preparing your evening meal.

The menus are divided into three sections: approximately 1,000 calories, 1,250 calories, and 1,500 calories daily. The lower calorie menus are suitable for women and the 1,500-calorie menus are mainly for men.

Special Diet Notes

1. As always, begin by deciding which daily calorie total will give you a satisfactory weight loss. You will find guidance on page 15.

2. Plan at least two or three days ahead, preferably one week ahead, and arrange your shopping so that you always have the right foods available.

3. Make sure that you eat a wide variety of foods to give a balanced healthy diet—select several different menus, preferably all different, each week.

4. Make up the Fiber-Filler for your daily allowance either daily or for several days in one batch, following the recipe on page 13.

5. Drink as much sugarless tea and coffee as you wish throughout the day, so long as you use only the skim milk from your daily allowance. Artificial sweeteners can be used. Water and drinks labeled ''low-calorie'' can also be drunk in unlimited quantities, but alcoholic drinks must be limited (see page 266).

1,000-Calorie Menu #1

	Calories	Fiber (g)
Daily allowance: Fiber-Filler, 1 cup skim milk, an orange, and an apple or pear	450	23.0
Breakfast Half portion of Fiber-Filler with milk from allowance Orange from allowance		
Lunch Banana and honey sandwich: 2 large thin slices of Arnold whole-wheat bread filled with 1 medium banana (mashed) and 2 teaspoons honey Apple or pear from allowance	235	5.1
Late afternoon Remaining Fiber-Filler with milk from allowance		
Evening meal * Stuffed Eggplant		

Mixed salad: 1 tomato (quartered), a
few sprigs of parsley, a few lettuce
leaves, ½ green pepper (chopped), 2
to 3 scallions (chopped), 1 tablespoon
oil-free French dressing
2 whole-wheat crackers spread with ¼
triangle Laughing Cow cheese,
topped with ½ sliced cucumber   397   11.6

Total	**1,082**	**39.7**

*STUFFED EGGPLANT   *Serves 2*

1   medium eggplant (¾ pound)
1   tablespoon diet margarine
1   small onion, chopped
2   medium tomatoes, chopped
1   large slice of Arnold whole-wheat bread
¼   cup skim milk (in addition to allowance)
2   (1-ounce) slices of lean boiled ham, chopped
     Generous pinch of dried mixed herbs
     Salt and pepper to taste
¼   cup grated Cheddar cheese

Preheat the oven to 350°F. Cut the eggplant in half lengthwise
and scoop out the flesh with a teaspoon. Chop the flesh. Heat
the margarine in a saucepan and fry the onion and tomatoes
gently for 5 minutes. Break up the bread, put in a bowl with
the milk, and let it soak for 5 minutes; squeeze dry and add to
the saucepan along with the ham and eggplant. Stir in the
herbs and season well with salt and pepper. Divide the mixture
in half and pile into the eggplant shells. Place in an ovenproof
dish and cover with foil. Bake in the oven for 1½ hours. Remove the foil and sprinkle with grated cheese. Return to the
oven for 15 minutes, until the cheese is melted and beginning
to brown. Serve hot.

1,000-Calorie Menu #2

	Calories	Fiber (g)
Daily allowance: Fiber-Filler, 1 cup skim milk, an orange, and an apple or pear	450	23.0
Breakfast Half portion of Fiber-Filler with milk from allowance		
Lunch Ham salad: 2 (1-ounce) slices of lean boiled ham with 1 medium tomato, 1 cup shredded Chinese cabbage, a small bunch of parsley, ⅔ cup grated carrot, and 1 large celery stalk, chopped		
Apple or pear from allowance	181	5.0
Late afternoon Remaining Fiber-Filler with milk from allowance		
Evening meal *Stuffed Flounder with Lemon and Shrimp Sauce 1 large broccoli stalk, boiled 1 large thin slice of Arnold whole-wheat bread spread with 1 teaspoon diet margarine		
Orange from allowance	377	9.1
Total	**1,008**	**37.1**

*STUFFED FLOUNDER WITH LEMON AND SHRIMP SAUCE *Serves 2*

STUFFING
¼ cup whole-wheat bread crumbs
1 small onion, peeled and finely chopped
2 carrots, peeled and finely grated
5 mushrooms, finely chopped
   Juice and rind of ½ lemon
   Pinch of lemon thyme
   Salt and pepper to taste
¾ pound fillet of flounder

SAUCE
1 tablespoon whole-wheat flour
1 tablespoon diet margarine
½ cup skim milk
1 tablespoon lemon juice
¼ pound shrimps
1 teaspoon chopped fresh parsley
   Salt and pepper to taste

Preheat the oven to 375°F. Mix the stuffing ingredients together. Spread the stuffing over the flounder and fold in half.
Place in an ovenproof dish, cover, and bake for 20 minutes, or
until the fish is tender. Meanwhile, prepare the sauce: Put the
flour, margarine, and milk in a saucepan and heat gently, stirring continuously, until it comes to a boil and thickens. Add
the lemon juice, shrimps, and parsley, and cook over low heat
for 5 minutes. Season. Arrange the stuffed fillets of flounder
on two serving plates and pour the sauce over the fish.

1,000-Calorie Menu #3

	Calories	Fiber (g)
Daily allowance: Fiber-Filler, 1 cup skim milk, an orange, and an apple or pear	450	23.0
Breakfast Half portion of Fiber-Filler with milk from allowance Orange from allowance		
Lunch 4 whole-wheat crackers, each spread with 1 tablespoon low-fat cottage cheese and topped with ½ medium sliced cucumber and 2 teaspoons corn relish Apple or pear from allowance	130	3.4
Late afternoon Remaining Fiber-Filler with milk from allowance		
Evening meal ½ cantaloupe or ¼ honeydew melon *Spinach and Cheese Soufflé 1 cup mixed vegetables	416	17.0
Total	**996**	**43.4**

*SPINACH AND CHEESE SOUFFLÉ   *Serves 2*

¾   cup finely chopped spinach
½   cup mashed potato
¼   cup grated Cheddar cheese

Salt and pepper to taste
2   tablespoons whole-wheat flour
1   tablespoon diet margarine
½   cup skim milk
2   eggs, separated

Preheat the oven to 425°F. Combine the spinach, potato, cheese, and salt and pepper in a bowl and mix thoroughly. Put the flour, margarine, and milk in a small saucepan and heat gently, stirring constantly, until the sauce thickens. Remove from the heat and beat in the egg yolks, then stir in the spinach mixture. Beat the egg whites until they form soft peaks and fold into the spinach mixture. Pour into a quart soufflé dish and bake in the oven for 25 to 30 minutes, or until it is golden brown and puffy. Serve immediately.

1,000-Calorie Menu #4

	Calories	Fiber (g)
Daily allowance: Fiber-Filler, 1 cup skim milk, an orange, and an apple or pear	450	23.0
Breakfast Half portion of Fiber-Filler with milk from allowance Orange from allowance		
Lunch Toasted cheese and date sandwich: Fill 2 large slices of Arnold whole-wheat bread with 2 tablespoons low-fat cottage cheese mixed with 2 chopped dates. Toast the sandwich on both sides, cut into quarters, and serve. Apple or pear from allowance	185	4.1

Late afternoon
Remaining Fiber-Filler with milk from
    allowance

Evening meal
*Minted Green Soup
2 whole-wheat crackers
1 chicken leg and thigh, broiled and skin
    removed, served hot or cold
*Kidney Bean, Onion, and Cauliflower
    Salad   433   16.7

	Total	1,068	43.8

*MINTED GREEN SOUP   *Serves 2*

4   large escarole leaves, rinsed and chopped
1   large cucumber, coarsely chopped
1   small onion, peeled and chopped
1   small potato, peeled and cut into four pieces
     Salt and pepper to taste
1   teaspoon chopped fresh mint
3   tablespoons low-fat natural yogurt

Put escarole, cucumber, onion, and potato in a medium saucepan with 1 cup water and bring to a boil. Reduce the heat and
simmer for 15 minutes. Let cool for a few minutes, then sieve
or purée in a blender. Season with salt and pepper, add the
mint and 2 tablespoons yogurt, and stir thoroughly. Chill in
the refrigerator. To serve, pour into two soup bowls and top
with remaining yogurt.

*KIDNEY BEAN, ONION, AND CAULIFLOWER
SALAD   *Serves 2*

⅔   cup canned red kidney beans, drained and rinsed
4   scallions, chopped
1½ cups raw cauliflower florets
¼   garlic clove, crushed
1   tablespoon oil-free French dressing
1   tablespoon lemon juice

Mix the kidney beans, scallions, and cauliflower in a salad
bowl. Mix the garlic with the French dressing and lemon juice
and pour over the vegetables. Toss well. Let stand for 10 minutes before serving.

1,000-Calorie Menu #5

	Calories	Fiber (g)
Daily allowance: Fiber-Filler, 1 cup skim milk, an orange, and an apple or pear	450	23
Breakfast Half portion of Fiber-Filler with milk from allowance Orange from allowance		
Lunch 4 whole-wheat crackers topped with ¼ cup cottage cheese mixed with 1 tablespoon raisins and 2 tablespoons chopped walnuts Apple or pear from allowance	227	3
Late afternoon Remaining Fiber-Filler with milk from allowance		

Evening meal
*Chicken Liver
½ cup fresh raspberries or ½ cup
   blueberries with 1 teaspoon sugar   334   18

                      Total   **1,011**   **44**

CHICKEN LIVER   Serves 2

1	teaspoon vegetable oil
½	cup brown rice
1	small onion, peeled and chopped
1	small red pepper, chopped
1	cup beef bouillon (made from 1 beef bouillon cube)
5	ounces chicken livers
¾	cup frozen peas, thawed
1	medium zucchini, thinly sliced, tossed with 1 to 2 tablespoons oil-free French dressing
1	teaspoon grated Parmesan cheese

Heat the oil in a medium-size saucepan and gently fry the rice, onion, and pepper for 3 to 4 minutes. Add the bouillon and bring to a boil. Reduce the heat and simmer for 25 minutes. Meanwhile, quickly brown the liver in a nonstick frying pan over medium heat. Add the liver and peas to the rice mixture and simmer for 10 to 15 minutes, or until the rice has absorbed most of the liquid. Arrange the zucchini slices around the edge of two serving plates and spoon the liver into the center. Sprinkle with Parmesan cheese.

1,250-Calorie Menu #1

	Calories	Fiber (g)
Daily allowance: Fiber-Filler, 1 cup skim milk, an orange, and an apple or pear	450	23.0

Breakfast
Half portion of Fiber-Filler with milk
  from allowance
Orange from allowance

Lunch
Liverwurst and lettuce sandwich: 2 large
  thin slices of Pepperidge Farm whole-
  wheat bread, filled with 2 tablespoons
  Underwood Liverwurst Spread and a
  thick layer of chopped lettuce
Apple or pear from allowance   234   3.1

Late afternoon
Remaining Fiber-Filler with milk from
  allowance

Evening meal
*Soufflé Omelet Filled with Shrimp,
  Corn, and Tomato
1 large broccoli stalk, boiled
2 small red-skinned potatoes, boiled
¼ cup portion vanilla ice cream with 1
  sliced medium banana   606   13.8
                                          ─────   ─────
                              Total   **1,290**   **39.9**

*SOUFFLÉ OMELET FILLED WITH SHRIMP, CORN,
AND TOMATO   *Serves 2*

FILLING
¾   cup (2 ounces) shrimps
¾   cup canned corn kernels
1   medium tomato, chopped
1   small onion, peeled and chopped
    Large pinch of oregano

OMELET
3　eggs, separated
　　Salt and pepper to taste
1　teaspoon vegetable oil
3　tablespoons grated cheddar cheese

Put the shrimp, corn, tomato, onion, and oregano in a sauce-pan, cover, and cook over medium heat for 10 to 15 minutes, or until the onion is soft. Prepare the omelet: Beat together the egg yolks, 2 tablespoons warm water, and salt and pepper. Beat the egg whites until they form soft peaks, then fold evenly into the beaten yolks. Heat the oil in a large frying pan or omelet pan and pour in the egg mixture, spreading it out evenly. Cook gently for 5 to 7 minutes, until the bottom is golden brown. Put under a preheated moderate broiler for 4 to 5 minutes, until the omelet is set and is lightly brown on the surface. Spoon the filling over half of the omelet, sprinkle with grated cheese, fold in half, and slice onto a hot plate. Cut into two portions and serve at once.

1,250-Calorie Menu #2

	Calories	Fiber (g)
Daily allowance: Fiber-Filler, 1 cup skim milk, an orange, and an apple or pear	450	23.0

Breakfast
Half portion of Fiber-Filler with milk
　from allowance
Orange from allowance

Lunch
4 whole-wheat crackers with 1 chopped
　hard-boiled egg mixed with 1
　tablespoon diet mayonnaise and salt

and pepper, topped with 2 chopped
lettuce leaves

Apple or pear from allowance	206	2.5

Late afternoon
Remaining Fiber-Filler with milk from
   allowance

Evening meal
*Chicken and Grapes with Mushroom
   Sauce
1 large potato, baked in its jacket (page
   20)
12 Brussels sprouts

½ cup fresh raspberries or blueberries with ½ cup plain low-fat yogurt	658	21.3
Total	**1,314**	**46.8**

*CHICKEN AND GRAPES WITH MUSHROOM SAUCE
Serves 2

2	chicken breast quarters with wing (7 ounces), skin removed
⅓	cup corn
10	mushrooms, sliced
½	cup dry white wine
½	cup chicken bouillon (made from ½ chicken bouillon cube)
	Salt and pepper to taste
2	tablespoons whole-wheat flour
1	tablespoon diet margarine
	Salt and pepper to taste
25	seedless grapes

Preheat the oven to 400°F. Put the chicken in an ovenproof dish with the corn, mushrooms, wine, bouillon, and salt and pepper. Cover and bake in the oven for 45 to 50 minutes, or until the chicken is tender. Remove the chicken to a serving dish and keep warm. Strain the bouillon into a saucepan; reserve the mushrooms and corn. To the bouillon add the flour, margarine, and salt and pepper. Stir over medium heat until it thickens. Add the grapes and corn and mushrooms, and mix thoroughly. Pour over the chicken and serve.

1,250-Calorie Menu #3

	Calories	Fiber (g)
Daily allowance: Fiber-Filler, 1 cup skim milk, an orange, and an apple or pear	450	23.0
Breakfast Half portion of Fiber-Filler with milk from allowance 1 large slice of Pepperidge Farm whole-wheat bread, toasted and spread with 1 teaspoon diet margarine and 2 teaspoons honey or marmalade	121	1.2
Lunch ½ cup fruit-flavored yogurt (blueberry, cherry, raspberry, etc.) 1 Nature Valley Granola Cluster (1 package) Apple or pear from allowance	281	3.1
Late afternoon Remaining Fiber-Filler with milk from allowance		

Evening meal
*Trout Kiev
1¼ cup peas and pearl onions
Orange from allowance   433   18.9

Total	**1,285**	**46.2**

*TROUT KIEV   *Serves 2*

2   (7-ounce) trout
2   teaspoons vegetable oil

STUFFING
⅓   cup canned corn
2   tablespoons slivered almonds
1   tablespoon diet margarine
1   garlic clove, crushed
2   tablespoons lemon juice

GARNISH
    Lemon slices
1   tablespoon toasted slivered almonds

Wipe the trout. Mix all the stuffing ingredients together and stuff the trout. Brush the skin with the oil and place on a broiler rack. Cook under the broiler for 8 to 10 minutes on each side, or until the fish is cooked through and the juices of the stuffing start to run out. Place on a hot serving dish and garnish with lemon slices and almonds.

1,250-Calorie Menu #4

	Calories	Fiber (g)
Daily allowance: Fiber-Filler, 1 cup skim milk, an orange, and an apple or pear	450	23.0

Breakfast
Half portion of Fiber-Filler with milk
    from allowance
Orange from allowance

Lunch
*Mushrooms on Toast
Apple or pear from allowance   230   4.8

Late afternoon
Remaining Fiber-Filler with milk from
    allowance

Evening meal
½ medium grapefruit
*Liver Stroganoff
1⅓ cups cauliflower florets, boiled
*Blueberry and Apple Fool   540   12.1
                                     _____
                          Total **1,220**   **39.9**

*MUSHROOMS ON TOAST   *Serves 2*

2   large slices of Pepperidge Farm whole-wheat bread
10   mushrooms, sliced
½   cup skim milk (in addition to allowance)
2   teaspoons cornstarch
     Dash of Worcestershire sauce
     Salt and pepper to taste
     A few sprigs of parsley

Toast the bread. Poach the mushrooms in skim milk for 5 minutes. Blend the cornstarch with a little cold water and stir into
the mushrooms. Bring to a boil, stirring, and cook for 2 minutes, until thickened. Add the Worcestershire sauce and salt
and pepper. Serve on toast, garnished with parsley.

*LIVER STROGANOFF *Serves 2*

1 teaspoon vegetable oil
7 ounces calf's liver, cut into thin strips
1 small onion, peeled and chopped
10 mushrooms, sliced
½ cup beef bouillon (made from ½ beef bouillon cube)
2 tablespoons dry sherry
3 tablespoons low-fat yogurt
1 cup green noodles, cooked and drained
   Chopped fresh parsley

Heat the oil in a medium-size saucepan, add the liver and onion, and fry gently for 3 to 4 minutes. Stir in the mushrooms, beef bouillon, and sherry; bring to a boil. Reduce the heat and simmer for 12 to 15 minutes, or until the liver is tender. Remove from heat and stir in 2 tablespoons yogurt. Arrange the noodles around the edges of two warmed plates and spoon the liver mixture into the center. Garnish with the remaining yogurt and the chopped parsley.

*BLUEBERRY AND APPLE FOOL *Serves 2*

1 cup blueberries
1 large cooking apple, cored and sliced
1 tablespoon sugar
1 cup plain low-fat yogurt

Cook the blueberries and apple with 4 tablespoons water in a covered pan until tender. Add the sugar. Purée the fruit in a blender and mix with the yogurt. Serve cold.

1,250-Calorie Menu #5

	Calories	Fiber (g)
Daily allowance: Fiber-Filler, 1 cup skim milk, an orange, and an apple or pear	450	23.0
Breakfast Half portion of Fiber-Filler with milk from allowance Orange from allowance		
Lunch 1 package of Lipton's Cup-a-Soup (chicken rice) 4 whole-wheat crackers topped with ¼ cup cottage cheese with chives and 2 sliced medium tomatoes Apple or pear from allowance	215	4.7
Late afternoon Remaining Fiber-Filler with milk from allowance		
Evening meal * Apricot-Stuffed Lamb Chops ¾ cup carrots, boiled 1 cup cabbage * Flambé Bananas	671	11.0
Total	**1,336**	**38.7**

*APRICOT-STUFFED LAMB CHOPS   *Serves 2*

2   (5-ounce) lean lamb loin chops

STUFFING
3   dried apricot halves, finely chopped
3   tablespoons whole-wheat bread crumbs
1   small onion, finely chopped
2   tablespoons finely chopped walnuts
1   egg white, beaten
⅛   teaspoon dried marjoram
    Salt and pepper to taste

Preheat the oven to 375°F. Using a sharp knife, cut a horizontal pocket in each chop from the fat edge toward the bone. Mix together all the stuffing ingredients. Fill the pockets with some of the stuffing. Form the remaining stuffing into small balls. Put the chops and stuffing balls in a shallow ovenproof dish. Cover and cook in the oven for 40 to 45 minutes, or until the lamb is tender and cooked through. Serve hot.

*FLAMBÉ BANANAS   *Serves 2*

2   medium bananas
3   tablespoons orange juice
1   teaspoon honey
¼   teaspoon ground cinnamon
1   tablespoon Grand Marnier or brandy
2   tablespoons chopped walnuts

Put the bananas in a medium-size saucepan or frying pan with the orange juice, honey, and cinnamon. Bring to a boil, reduce the heat, and simmer gently for 3 to 4 minutes, or until the bananas are tender. Place with the juice on a serving dish. Heat the Grand Marnier and set aflame. While flaming, pour over the bananas, and let flames die out. Sprinkle with chopped walnuts.

1,250-Calorie Menu #6

	Calories	Fiber (g)
Daily allowance: Fiber-Filler, 1 cup skim milk, an orange, and an apple or pear	450	23.0
Breakfast Half-portion of Fiber-Filler with milk from allowance Orange from allowance		
Lunch Banana, raisin, and almond sandwich: 2 large slices of whole-wheat bread filled with 1 medium banana mashed with 2 teaspoons honey and mixed with 2 tablespoons raisins and 1 teaspoon slivered almonds Apple or pear from allowance	338	7.3
Late afternoon Remaining Fiber-Filler with milk from allowance		
Evening meal *Crab and Apple Cocktail 5 ounces ham steak, broiled, with 1 large juice-packed pineapple ring, heated through under the broiler ⅔ cup broccoli, cooked ½ cup green beans, cooked	546	11.1
Total	**1,334**	**41.4**

CRAB AND APPLE COCKTAIL *Serves 2*

1   (3-ounce) can of crab meat, flaked
1   medium eating apple (in addition to allowance), cored
     and chopped
¼   cup canned corn

DRESSING
1   teaspoon tomato purée
2   teaspoons diet mayonnaise
⅛   teaspoon dry mustard
1   teaspoon lemon juice
1   teaspoon skim milk
     A few lettuce leaves, shredded
1   medium tomato, sliced
     Lemon wedges

Put the crab, apple, and corn in a medium-size bowl and mix
well. Mix all the dressing ingredients and stir into the crab
mixture. Line two glass dishes with shredded lettuce and pile
the crab and apple mixture on top. Garnish with the tomato
and lemon. Chill.

1,250-Calorie Menu #7

	Calories	Fiber (g)
Daily allowance: Fiber-Filler, 1 cup skim milk, an orange, and an apple or pear	450	23.0

Breakfast
Whole portion of Fiber-Filler with milk
   from allowance

Lunch
Creamed mushrooms on toast: 1 large
   slice of whole-wheat bread, toasted
   and topped with whole package Birds

Eye Green Peas with Cream Sauce,
heated and mixed with 2½
tablespoons bran and 1 teaspoon
Worcestershire sauce
Apple or pear from allowance   213   6.8

Late afternoon
1 Nature Valley Granola Bar
Orange from allowance   150   1.0

Evening meal
*Tropical Melon
*Chicken and Fruit Salad
4 whole-wheat crackers spread with 1
   teaspoon margarine   488   7.1
                                               _____
                            Total   1,301   37.9

*TROPICAL MELON   *Serves 2*

3   cups watermelon balls
1   tablespoon white rum
1   tablespoon orange juice
2   teaspoons shredded coconut

Put the melon balls in a mixing bowl with the rum and orange
juice and mix well. Cover and let stand for 1 hour in a cool
place. Divide equally between two glass dishes and sprinkle
with the coconut. Serve chilled.

*CHICKEN AND FRUIT SALAD   *Serves 2*

1   (7-ounce) chicken breast, skinned and diced
½   cup juice-packed crushed pineapple
25 seedless green grapes, halved
½   cup low-fat yogurt

1   tablespoon lemon juice
     Salt and pepper to taste
     A few lettuce leaves
1   cucumber, sliced
¾   cup canned corn

Put the chicken, pineapple, and grapes in a bowl. Mix the
yogurt with the lemon juice and season well with salt and pepper. Stir into the chicken mixture. Arrange a bed of lettuce
leaves on two plates; divide the chicken and fruit salad equally
between the two plates and pile into the center. Arrange a ring
of cucumber slices around the edge and then spoon a thin ring
of corn on top of the cucumber slices.

1,250-Calorie Menu #8

	Calories	Fiber (g)
Daily allowance: Fiber-Filler, 1 cup skim milk, an orange, and an apple or pear	450	23.0
Breakfast Half portion of Fiber-Filler with milk from allowance 1 medium banana	85	2.7
Lunch ¾ cup canned baked beans in tomato sauce, heated and topped with 1 tablespoon grated Swiss cheese Orange from allowance	251	23.0
Late afternoon Remaining Fiber-Filler with milk from allowance		

Evening meal
*Steak Kebabs
Green salad: a few lettuce leaves, a few
   slices of cucumber, a small bunch of
   parsley
Apple or pear from allowance   522   8.5

                    Total   **1,308**   **57.2**

*STEAK KEBABS   *Serves 2*

MARINADE
1   tablespoon vegetable oil
2   tablespoons red wine
1   tablespoon diet mayonnaise

½   pound lean chuck steak, cut into cubes
6   small white onions
8   cherry tomatoes
6   fresh mushroom caps
1   small green pepper, seeded and cubed
6   bay leaves

1   cup cooked brown rice
⅓   cup canned corn, heated

Mix the marinade ingredients together. Put the cubes of steak in the marinade and leave, covered, for approximately 1 hour. Then thread the steak on two long or four medium skewers, alternating with the onions, tomatoes, mushrooms, green pepper, and bay leaves. Cook under a preheated broiler for 15 minutes, turning several times and brushing with the marinade. Mix the rice with the corn and spoon onto a warm serving dish. Place the kebabs on top and serve.

1,250-Calorie Menu #9

	Calories	Fiber (g)
Daily allowance: Fiber-Filler, 1 cup skim milk, an orange, and an apple or pear	450	23.0
Breakfast Whole portion of Fiber-Filler with milk from allowance		
Lunch Mushroom scramble on toast: Poach ½ cup sliced mushrooms in ¼ cup skim milk (in addition to allowance) in a saucepan. Add 2 eggs, beaten with salt and pepper, and cook gently, stirring, until the eggs are creamy. Serve on 1 large slice of Arnold whole-wheat bread, toasted. Orange from allowance	248	2.4
Late afternoon 1 small (½-ounce) package of potato chips Apple or pear from allowance	80	1.0
Evening meal *Ham with Bean Salad *Fruited Orange Sorbet	555	21.8
Total	**1,333**	**48.2**

*HAM WITH BEAN SALAD   Serves 2

5   (1-ounce) slices of lean boiled ham
½   cup green beans, frozen
2   large celery stalks, chopped
1   onion, finely chopped
1   cup canned kidney beans, drained
1   small green pepper, seeded and sliced
4   tablespoons oil-free French dressing
      Salt and pepper to taste
      Chopped lettuce

Remove all visible fat from the meat. Cook the green beans in salted water until just tender, drain, and let cool. Cut them into bite-size pieces and mix in a salad bowl with the celery, onion, kidney beans, and green pepper. Add the dressing and salt and pepper and mix well. Serve the salad with the sliced ham on a bed of lettuce.

*FRUITED ORANGE SORBET   Serves 2

½   cup orange juice
2   tablespoons sugar
2   tablespoons raisins
1   large orange
1   egg white

Put the orange juice, sugar, and raisins in a saucepan and heat until the sugar dissolves. Let cool. Cut the orange in half and scoop out the flesh, reserving the two halves of orange peel. Purée the orange flesh in a blender and stir into the orange juice. Pour into a freezer container and freeze until crystals form. Beat with a fork. Beat the egg white until it forms soft peaks, then fold in the orange mixture. Return to the freezer until frozen. To serve, spoon into the orange-peel shells.

1,500-Calorie Menu #1

	Calories	Fiber (g)
Daily allowance: Fiber-Filler, 1 cup skim milk, an orange, and an apple or pear	450	23.0
Breakfast Half portion of Fiber-Filler with milk from allowance 1 egg, boiled 1 large slice of whole-wheat bread spread with 1 teaspoon diet margarine	172	1.2
Lunch Cheese and pineapple on toast: 1 large slice of Pepperidge Farm whole-wheat bread, toasted and covered with ¼ cup grated Cheddar cheese and 1 juice-packed pineapple ring. Heat through under a broiler until cheese has melted. Garnish with a few sprigs of parsley. Apple or pear from allowance	237	2.2
Late afternoon Remaining Fiber-Filler with milk from allowance		
Evening meal *Tuna Pies *Orange and Watercress Salad ½ cup plain low-fat yogurt with 1 medium banana, sliced	612	14.2
Total	**1,471**	**40.6**

*TUNA PIES   *Serves 2*

PASTRY
¾   cup whole-wheat flour
     Pinch of salt
¼   cup diet margarine

FILLING
½   cup water-packed tuna, drained and flaked
3   tablespoons grated Cheddar cheese
1   teaspoon tomato purée
1   teaspoon diet mayonnaise
1   medium tomato, chopped
1   medium apple (in addition to allowance), cored and
     chopped
     Pepper to taste

¼   teaspoon salt in 3 tablespoons warm water

Preheat the oven to 400°F. Put the flour and salt in a bowl and cut in the margarine until the mixture resembles bread crumbs. Mix in enough cold water to form a soft dough, lightly knead, then cut in two. Roll out each half to a 7-inch circle. Mix all the filling ingredients together. Divide the filling equally between the two pastry circles. Bring up the edges to meet in the middle to form a turnover shape. Flute the joined edges, using a finger and a thumb. Place on a baking sheet and brush with the salt and water. Bake in the oven for 25 to 30 minutes, or until golden brown. Serve hot or cold.

*ORANGE AND WATERCRESS SALAD   *Serves 2*

2   medium oranges (1 orange from allowance)
     Large bunch of watercress
2   tablespoons lemon juice

Salt and pepper to taste
A few lettuce leaves

Peel and section oranges. Divide the watercress into sprigs and mix with the orange segments, lemon juice, and seasoning. Line two individual salad bowls with lettuce leaves and spoon in the orange and watercress salad.

1,500-Calorie Menu #2

	Calories	Fiber (g)
Daily allowance: Fiber-Filler, 1 cup skim milk, an orange, and an apple or pear	450	23.0
Breakfast		
Half portion of Fiber-Filler with milk from allowance		
1 large slice of whole-wheat bread, toasted and spread with 1 teaspoon diet margarine and 2 teaspoons honey or marmalade	134	1.2
Lunch		
1 whole-wheat roll, split and filled with 1 chopped hard-boiled egg mixed with 1 tablespoon diet mayonnaise, topped with chopped lettuce		
1 Crown Pilot Cracker		
Apple or pear from allowance	308	3.2
Late afternoon		
Remaining Fiber-Filler with milk from allowance		
Evening meal		
*Vegetable and Ham Gougère		
*Ice Cream and Orange Sundae	585	19.3
Total	**1,477**	**46.7**

*VEGETABLE AND HAM GOUGÈRE   *Serves 2*

FILLING
1   cup canned lima beans
2   tablespoons peas, cooked
1   cup cauliflower florets, cooked
1   large carrot, sliced and cooked
5   fresh mushrooms, sliced
2   (1-ounce) slices of boiled ham, chopped
2   tablespoons whole-wheat flour
2   tablespoons diet margarine
¾   cup skim milk
     Salt and pepper to taste
2   tablespoons grated Cheddar cheese

CHOUX PASTRY
⅓   cup water
3   tablespoons diet margarine
¼   cup whole-wheat flour
1   egg, beaten

Preheat the oven to 425°F. Put the lima beans, peas, cauliflower, carrot, mushrooms, and ham in a bowl and mix well. Put the flour, margarine, milk, and salt and pepper in a small pan. Stir over low heat until it thickens. Add the vegetable and ham mixture and mix thoroughly. Pour into a 1-quart ovenproof dish and sprinkle with the grated cheese. To make the pastry, put water and margarine in a small saucepan; bring to a boil. Stir in the flour all at once and beat well until the mixture leaves the sides of the pan. Remove from the heat and gradually beat in the egg. Using a ½-inch nozzle, pipe the choux pastry around the edge of the filling. Bake in the hot oven for 15 minutes, then reduce the heat to 375°F and cook for 15 minutes, or until the cheese is beginning to brown. Serve hot.

*ICE CREAM AND ORANGE SUNDAE   *Serves 2*

½   cup vanilla ice cream
2   medium oranges (1 from allowance), sectioned
1   tablespoon Country Morning granola with almonds and
      dates

Layer the ice cream with the orange segments in dessert dishes
and sprinkle with granola.

1,500-Calorie Menu #3

	Calories	Fiber (g)
Daily allowance: Fiber-Filler, 1 cup skim milk, an orange, and an apple or pear	450	23.0
Breakfast Whole portion of Fiber-Filler with milk from allowance		
Lunch Cottage cheese and coleslaw salad: ½ cup low-fat cottage cheese, served with 1 cup coleslaw and 1 medium tomato, quartered Orange from allowance	222	6.5
Late afternoon 1 small (¾-ounce) package of corn chips Apple or pear from allowance	114	1.0
Evening meal ½ grapefruit *Ham Steaks with Somerset Sauce ¾ cup lima beans, cooked 1½ cups cauliflower, cooked		

4 whole-wheat crackers with 3 tablespoons cream cheese		
1 large celery stalk	712	15.3
Total	**1,498**	**45.8**

*HAM STEAKS WITH SOMERSET SAUCE   *Serves 2*

4   (1-ounce) ham steaks

SAUCE
⅓   cup apple cider vinegar and 4 tablespoons water
1   small apple (in addition to allowance), cored and chopped
2   tablespoons raisins
4   cloves
¼   teaspoon dry mustard
1   teaspoon cornstarch blended with 1 teaspoon water

8   slices of red apple (in addition to allowance), dipped in lemon juice

Make cuts in the fat of the ham steaks to prevent curling during cooking. Broil 8 to 10 minutes on each side, or until the fat is well browned. Meanwhile, put the sauce ingredients in a medium-size saucepan and bring to a boil, stirring constantly until thickened. Arrange ham steaks on a serving dish and spoon the sauce over them. Garnish with apple slices.

1,500-Calorie Menu #4

	Calories	Fiber (g)
Daily allowance: Fiber-Filler, 1 cup skim milk, an orange, and an apple or pear	450	23

Breakfast
Whole portion of Fiber-Filler with milk from allowance

Lunch

Cottage cheese and carrot sandwich: 2
   large slices of whole-wheat bread
   filled with ¼ cup cottage cheese with
   chives mixed with ⅔ cup grated
   carrot   258   4

Late afternoon

1 Nature Valley Coconut Granola Bar
Orange from allowance   120   1

Evening meal

1 chicken leg and thigh, baked in the
   oven, skin removed
1 large baked potato (page 20), split and
   topped with 1 tablespoon cottage
   cheese with chives mixed with 2
   tablespoons oil-free French dressing
¾ cup frozen mixed vegetables
*Lemon Cheesecake   690   10

	Total	**1,518**	**38**

*LEMON CHEESECAKE   Serves 2

2   graham crackers, crushed
1   tablespoon diet margarine, melted

FILLING

¼   cup low-fat cottage cheese, sieved
2   level tablespoons sugar
1   egg, separated
    Juice and grated rind of ¼ lemon
2   teaspoons unflavored gelatin
¼   cup low-fat yogurt

2   kiwi fruit, peeled and sliced

Combine crumbs and margarine. Divide equally between two individual glass dishes; press down well. Leave in a cool place. Beat together the cottage cheese, sugar, and egg yolk until smooth. Add the lemon juice and rind. Dissolve the gelatin in 2 tablespoons water in a double boiler. Stir into the cheese mixture, along with the yogurt. Beat the egg white until it forms soft peaks, then fold into the other ingredients and pour over the crumb crust. Refrigerate. Decorate with kiwi fruit slices.

1,500-Calorie Menu #5

	Calories	Fiber (g)
Daily allowance: Fiber-Filler, 1 cup skim milk, an orange, and an apple or pear	450	23.0
Breakfast Whole portion of Fiber-Filler with milk from allowance		
Lunch *Minestrone 1 piece of whole-wheat matzo spread with 1 teaspoon diet margarine Apple or pear from allowance	383	10.0
Late afternoon 1 large slice of Pepperidge Farm whole-wheat bread spread with 1 teaspoon diet margarine and 2 teaspoons honey Orange from allowance	121	1.5

Evening meal
5 ounces rump steak, grilled and all fat
    trimmed off
Mixed salad: a few lettuce leaves, ½
    cucumber (sliced), 1 medium tomato
    (sliced), ½ green pepper (sliced), ½
    onion, and 1 tablespoon oil-free
    French dressing
* Strawberry Sundae   598   8.0

	Total	**1,552**	**42.5**

*MINESTRONE   Serves 2

1   large onion, coarsely grated or finely chopped
1⅓ cups coarsely grated carrot
1⅓ cups coarsely grated parsnip
1   chicken bouillon cube
1   cup tomato juice
½   cup whole-wheat macaroni
1   cup finely shredded cabbage
    Salt and pepper to taste
1   tablespoon chopped fresh parsley
2   tablespoons grated Parmesan cheese

Put the onion, carrot, and parsnip in a saucepan. Dissolve the chicken bouillon cube in 1 cup boiling water and add to the vegetables in the pan with the tomato juice and macaroni. Bring to a boil, stir well, cover, and simmer gently for 15 minutes. Add the cabbage, bring back to a boil, and cook, covered, for a further 5 to 10 minutes, until the cabbage is tender. Season with salt and pepper and stir in the chopped parsley. Serve in two soup bowls and sprinkle the cheese on top.

*STRAWBERRY SUNDAE   *Serves 2*

JELLY
1   cup strawberries
1   tablespoon brown sugar
2   teaspoons powdered gelatin, dissolved in 2 tablespoons
    water

TOPPING
¼   cup Cool Whip
3   tablespoons plain low-fat yogurt
2   teaspoons sugar

Put the strawberries, sugar, and ¾ cup water in a small saucepan and bring to a boil. Reduce the heat and simmer gently for
2 to 3 minutes. Remove from the heat and let cool for a few
minutes. Stir in the dissolved gelatin and pour into two sundae
glasses. Leave to set, tilted so that gelatin sets at an angle.
Meanwhile, blend the Cool Whip, yogurt, and sugar. When
the strawberry gelatin is set, spoon half the topping into each
glass, on top of the gelatin. Serve at once.

Canned and Packaged F-Plan

As the title suggests, these menus contain a large number of canned and packaged convenience foods for those whose lifestyle leaves little time or inclination for food preparation. While they follow most of the basic F-Plan diet rules, the daily allowance has been adjusted so that packaged cereals can be used in place of Fiber-Filler, to cut out the need to weigh out and make up the ingredients. Adequate food storage space, especially a freezer, is an advantage when following these menus unless you can shop frequently.

To enable both men and women to use these menus, a choice of menus providing approximately 1,000 calories, 1,250 calories, and 1,500 calories daily has been given. All you have to do is to decide which daily calorie total will suit you best (give you the most satisfactory weight loss). You could find that if you are strict from Monday to Friday, selecting menus from the 1,000-calorie section, you will be able to allow yourself to be a little more liberal on weekends and choose menus from the 1,250-calorie or 1,500-calorie section, and still achieve a satisfactory weight loss.

If you find that you long for the occasional alcoholic drink or bar of chocolate and can stick to a diet only if it allows you to indulge occasionally, turn to the 1,500-calorie menus. However, it may be necessary to limit strictly the number of days when you allow yourself an intake of 1,500 calories if your weight loss is slow.

Special Diet Notes

1. Select the menus for at least one week at a time so that you can plan the shopping and always have the right foods available.

2. The daily allowance for all the 1,000-calorie and 1,250-calorie menus includes ⅔ cup Bran Buds in place of Fiber-Filler. The 1,500-calorie menus have a high-fiber breakfast

cereal with dried fruit for breakfast, and no Fiber-Filler has been included in the daily allowance.

3. All the menus include 1 cup skim milk and two whole fresh fruits (an orange and an apple or pear) in the daily allowance.

4. Use your skim milk allowance with the Bran Buds or cereal and in tea and coffee.

5. Tea and coffee are unlimited so long as you don't add sugar (artificial sweeteners can be used). In addition, you can drink unlimited amounts of those drinks labeled "low-calorie," and water.

6. The menus are divided into breakfast, a light meal, a main meal, and an anytime snack or drink. You can eat these meals in any order you wish throughout the day, but eat *only* those meals/snacks and/or drinks included in your chosen menu.

1,000-Calorie Menu #1

	Calories	Fiber (g)
Daily allowance: ⅔ cup Bran Buds, 1 cup skim milk, an orange, and an apple or pear	421	24.0
Breakfast Half portion of Bran Buds with milk from allowance		
Light meal 1 Cup Progresso Lentil Soup 1 whole-wheat matzo Apple or pear from allowance	265	7.5
Main meal 1 (9-ounce) package of Green Giant Steak and Green Pepper in Sauce with Rice and Vegetable Orange from allowance	250	2.0

Snacks
Remaining Bran Buds with milk from
    allowance
1 Fibermed Apple/Currant Biscuit   60   5.0

Total	**996**	**38.5**

1,000-Calorie Menu #2

	Calories	Fiber (g)
Daily allowance: ⅔ cup Bran Buds, 1 cup skim milk, an orange, and an apple or pear	421	24

Breakfast
⅓ cup Bran Buds with milk from
    allowance
Orange from allowance

Light meal
2 large slices of Arnold whole-wheat
    bread filled with 2 tablespoons
    Underwood Chicken Spread
Chopped lettuce
1 medium carrot, cut into sticks   207   5

Main meal
2 (1-ounce) slices of corned beef
1 cup coleslaw
Mixed salad: a few lettuce leaves, ½
    cucumber (sliced), 1 medium tomato
    (sliced), 2 scallions (chopped), ½
    green pepper (chopped), with 1
    tablespoon oil-free French dressing
4 whole-wheat crackers spread with 1
    teaspoon diet margarine   380   10

Snacks
Remaining Bran Buds with milk from
    allowance
Apple or pear from allowance

| | | Total | 1,008 | 39 |

1,000-Calorie Menu #3

	Calories	Fiber (g)
Daily allowance: ⅔ cup Bran Buds, 1 cup skim milk, an orange, and an apple or pear	421	24.0
Breakfast Half portion of Bran Buds with milk from allowance 1 large slice of Pepperidge Farm whole-wheat bread, toasted and spread with 1 teaspoon diet margarine	81	1.2
Light meal 1 large slice of whole-wheat bread, toasted and topped with ½ cup canned baked beans in tomato sauce	215	13.7
Main meal 1 (9-ounce) package of boil-in-bag Green Giant Beef Stew 9 frozen Brussels sprouts, cooked ¼ cup canned corn Orange from allowance	310	4.6
Snacks Remaining Bran Buds with milk from allowance Apple or pear from allowance		
Total	1,027	43.5

1,000-Calorie Menu #4

	Calories	Fiber (g)
Daily allowance: ⅔ cup Bran Buds, 1 cup skim milk, an orange, and an apple or pear	421	24
Breakfast Bran Buds with milk from allowance		
Light meal 4 whole-wheat crackers, spread with 2 tablespoons Underwood Chicken Spread and topped with a sliced tomato and chopped lettuce Apple or pear from allowance	162	4
Main meal 1 (11-ounce) package of Stouffer's Lean Cuisine frozen Zucchini Lasagna ¾ cup frozen peas, boiled 1 medium banana	433	12
Snack Orange from allowance		
Total	**1,016**	**40**

1,000-Calorie Menu #5

	Calories	Fiber (g)
Daily allowance: ⅔ cup Bran Buds, 1 cup skim milk, an orange, and an apple or pear	421	24.0

Breakfast
Bran Buds with milk from allowance

Light meal
½ cup cottage cheese with chives
1 cup coleslaw
Apple or pear from allowance   201   5.0

Main meal
1 (9½-ounce) can of Campbell's
   Chunky Split Pea and Ham Soup
1 Fibermed biscuit
Orange from allowance   358   10.0

Snacks
1 medium carrot, cut into sticks
1 large celery stalk   24   1.9

	Total	**1,004**	**40.9**

1,000-Calorie Menu #6

	Calories	**Fiber (g)**

Daily allowance: ⅔ cup Bran Buds, 1
   cup skim milk, an orange, and an
   apple or pear   421   24.0

Breakfast
Half portion of Bran Buds with milk
   from allowance

Light meal
½ cup Dannon fruit-flavored low-fat
   yogurt
1 Carnation Chocolate Crunch Breakfast
   Bar
Orange from allowance   245   1.0

Main meal
1 egg, poached
1 slice of Canadian bacon
¾ cup canned baked beans in tomato
    sauce
Apple or pear from allowance   293   12.5

Snacks
Remaining Bran Buds with milk from
    allowance
2 whole-wheat crackers spread with 1
    tablespoon Featherweight Low
    Calorie Strawberry Preserves   59   0.9

	Total	**1,018**	**38.4**

1,000-Calorie Menu #7

	Calories	**Fiber (g)**
Daily allowance: ⅔ cup Bran Buds, 1 cup skim milk, an orange, and an apple or pear	421	24.0

Breakfast
Half portion of Bran Buds with milk
    from allowance

Light meal
1 cup Progresso Lentil Soup
4 whole-wheat crackers
Apple or pear from allowance   214   7.0

Main meal
1 package of Lean Cuisine Fillet of Fish
¾ cup Birds Eye Corn Jubilee   360   7.0
Orange from allowance

Snacks
Remaining Bran Buds with milk from
    allowance
2 large celery stalks   6   0.6

	Total	**1,001**	**38.6**

1,250-Calorie Menu #1

	Calories	Fiber (g)

Daily allowance: ⅔ cup Bran Buds, 1 cup
    skim milk, an orange, and an apple or
    pear   421   24.0

Breakfast
Bran Buds with milk from allowance

Light meal
Peanut salad sandwich: 2 large slices of
    Pepperidge Farm whole-wheat bread
    spread with 2 tablespoons peanut
    butter and filled with chopped lettuce,
    1 tomato (sliced), and a few
    cucumber slices
Orange from allowance   358   6.8

Main meal
1 (7½-ounce) can of Dinty Moore Beef
    Stew
¾ cup Americana Pennsylvania Dutch
    Style vegetables
¾ cup Birds Eye Corn Jubilee   348   9.8

Snacks
1 Fibermed Apple/Currant Biscuit
    spread with 1 tablespoon
    Featherweight Strawberry Preserves
Apple or pear from allowance   87   5.0

| | Total | 1,214 | 45.6 |

1,250-Calorie Menu #2

	Calories	Fiber (g)
Daily allowance: ⅔ cup Bran Buds, 1 cup skim milk, an orange, and an apple or pear	421	24.0

Breakfast
Bran Buds with milk from allowance
Orange from allowance

Light meal
1 large slice of Arnold whole-wheat
    bread topped with 2 tablespoons
    grated Cheddar cheese mixed with 2
    tablespoons sweet pickle relish,
    broiled until cheese melts
2 medium tomatoes, sliced
Apple or pear from allowance   198   4.2

Main meal
1 (8-ounce) Morton Beef Pie
¾ cup frozen peas, boiled
½ cup fruit-flavored low-fat yogurt   538   9.8

Snack ·
1 Fibermed Apple/Currant Biscuit   60   5.0

| | Total | 1,217 | 43.0 |

1,250-Calorie Menu #3

	Calories	Fiber (g)
Daily allowance: ⅔ cup Bran Buds, 1 cup skim milk, an orange, and an apple or pear	421	24.0
Breakfast Bran Buds with milk from allowance		
Light meal 1 (10-ounce) can of Campbell's Split Pea with Ham and Bacon Soup 4 whole-wheat crackers Apple or pear from allowance	287	11.7
Main meal 1 (7-ounce) Weight Watchers Sausage and Cheese Pizza Salad: a few lettuce leaves, 1 tomato (sliced), ½ cucumber (sliced), 1 green pepper (sliced), with 1 tablespoon low-calorie oil-free French dressing ½ cup juice-packed peach slices	531	7.6
Snacks Orange from allowance Fibermed Apple/Currant Biscuit	60	5.0
Total	**1,299**	**48.3**

1,250-Calorie Menu #4

	Calories	Fiber (g)
Daily allowance: ⅔ cup Bran Buds, 1 cup skim milk, an orange, and an apple or pear	421	24.0
Breakfast Bran Buds with milk from allowance		
Light meal Bacon and green pepper sandwich: 2 slices of whole-wheat bread filled with 2 tablespoons Underwood Liverwurst Spread and 1 chopped green pepper Orange from allowance	231	3.2
Main meal 1 McDonald's Quarter Pounder ½ cup chickpeas (from salad bar) ½ cup mushrooms (from salad bar) ½ cup fruit-flavored low-fat yogurt	513	8.5
Snacks Apple or pear from allowance 1 Fibermed Apple/Currant Biscuit	60	5.0
Total	**1,225**	**40.7**

1,250-Calorie Menu #5

	Calories	Fiber (g)
Daily allowance: ⅔ cup Bran Buds, 1 cup skim milk, an orange, and an apple or pear	421	24.0
Breakfast Bran Buds with milk from allowance		
Light meal Creamy mushrooms on toast: 1 large slice of Pepperidge Farm whole-wheat bread, toasted and topped with 6 ounces Green Giant frozen Mushrooms in Butter Sauce, mixed with 1 tablespoon bran and 1 teaspoon Worcestershire sauce and heated through ½ Nature Valley Honey 'N Oats Granola Bar Apple or pear from allowance	252	6.5
Main meal 2 Oscar Mayer Smoked Breakfast Sausages ¾ cup Birds Eye Frozen Succotash ¾ cup Progresso Blackeyed Peas, heated ½ cup plain low-fat yogurt with 1 teaspoon honey or brown sugar	411	10.0
Snacks ½ cup chocolate ice cream Orange from allowance	148	0.0
Total	**1,232**	**40.5**

1,250-Calorie Menu #6

	Calories	Fiber (g)
Daily allowance: ⅔ cup Bran Buds, 1 cup skim milk, an orange, and an apple or pear	421	24.0
Breakfast Half portion of Bran Buds with milk from allowance		
1 egg, poached, on a large slice of toasted whole-wheat bread	133	1.2
Light meal 1½ sardines in tomato sauce ½ cup three-bean salad A few lettuce leaves 1 medium tomato, sliced Apple or pear from allowance	365	16.0
Main meal 1 (9-ounce) package of Green Giant Steak and Green Peppers in Sauce with Rice and Vegetable ½ cup green beans, cooked ½ cup canned corn, cooked Orange from allowance	340	6.7
Snack Remaining Bran Buds with milk from allowance		
Total	**1,259**	**47.9**

1,250-Calorie Menu #7

	Calories	Fiber (g)
Daily allowance: ⅔ cup Bran Buds, 1 cup skim milk, an orange, and an apple or pear	421	24.0
Breakfast Half portion of Bran Buds with milk from allowance 1 large slice of Arnold whole-wheat bread, toasted and spread with 1 teaspoon diet margarine and 1 teaspoon honey or marmalade	91	1.2
Light meal ½ Weight Watchers Sausage and Cheese Pizza ¼ cup canned baked beans in tomato sauce mixed with 1 tablespoon bran Orange from allowance	279	8.3
Main meal Mushroom omelet: Beat 2 eggs with 2 tablespoons water, salt and pepper, and a pinch of oregano. Cook in a nonstick omelet pan and fill with 2 ounces Green Giant Mushrooms in Butter Sauce. ½ cup canned corn, heated ¼ cup plain low-fat yogurt spooned over 1 sliced unpeeled cored fresh pear (in addition to allowance)	416	10.0
Snacks Remaining Bran Buds with milk from allowance Apple or pear from allowance		
Total	**1,207**	**43.5**

1,500-Calorie Menu #1

	Calories	Fiber (g)
Daily allowance: 1 cup skim milk, an orange, and an apple or pear	276	8.2
Breakfast 1 cup Kellogg's All-Bran with 2 tablespoons raisins and milk from allowance	187	18.2
Light meal 1 (7-ounce) can of Franco-American spaghetti with tomato and cheese sauce 1 Crunchola peanut butter and chocolate chip bar 1 medium banana	415	4.7
Main meal 1 (10-ounce) package of Green Giant Chicken and Vegetables ½ cup chickpeas Orange from allowance	356	4.0
Snacks Apple or pear from allowance 4 whole-wheat crackers spread with 2 tablespoons Underwood Chicken Spread and topped with ½ sweet pickle	226	2.6
Total	**1,460**	**37.7**

1,500-Calorie Menu #2

	Calories	Fiber (g)
Daily allowance: 1 cup skim milk, an orange, and an apple or pear	276	8.2
Breakfast ½ cup Kellogg's All-Bran with 1 tablespoon chopped dried apricots and milk from allowance	126	14.6
Light meal 1 (12¾-ounce) package of Lean Cuisine Chicken and Vegetables with Vermicelli ½ cup canned kidney beans Apple or pear from allowance	394	15.8
Main meal ½ (10-ounce) package of Mrs. Paul's Fish au Gratin ¾ cup frozen peas, boiled ½ cup juice-packed peach slices, topped with ¼ cup vanilla ice cream and ⅓ cup Kellogg's Cracklin' Bran	594	14.2
Snack and drinks Orange from allowance 1½ ounces (1 jigger) gin, rum, vodka, or whiskey with low-calorie mixers or other drinks chosen from chart (page 266) to the value of 110 calories	110	0.0
Total	**1,500**	**52.8**

1,500-Calorie Menu #3

	Calories	Fiber (g)
Daily allowance: 1 cup skim milk, an orange, and an apple or pear	276	8.2
Breakfast ¾ cup Kellogg's All-Bran with 1 tablespoon raisins and milk from allowance	125	13.3
Light meal 1 cup Progresso Lentil Soup 4 whole-wheat crackers Apple or pear from allowance	214	6.7
Main meal 1 (11-ounce) package of Lean Cuisine Zucchini Lasagna ½ cup three-bean salad 1 large juice-packed pineapple ring topped with ½ cup yogurt and 4 Kellogg's Frosted Mini Wheats, crushed	606	21.3
Snacks and drinks Drink(s) from chart (page 266) to value of 160 calories 1 small (¾-ounce) package of potato chips Orange from allowance	274	1.0
Total	**1,495**	**50.5**

1,500-Calorie Menu #4

	Calories	Fiber (g)
Daily allowance: 1 cup skim milk, an orange, and an apple or pear	276	8.2
Breakfast ¾ cup Kellogg's All-Bran with 1 tablespoon chopped dried apricots and milk from allowance	126	14.6
Light meal Tuna salad sandwich: 2 slices of Pepperidge Farm whole-wheat bread filled with ½ cup water-packed tuna, 1 tablespoon mayonnaise, lettuce, 1 sliced tomato, and a few slices of cucumber 1 Fibermed Apple/Currant Biscuit Orange from allowance	411	10.3
Main meal 1 (8-ounce) Morton Chicken Pot Pie, cooked ½ cup (whole package) Birds Eye Succotash, cooked 1 medium banana	515	6.3
Snacks Apple or pear from allowance 1 roll Nature Valley Raisin Granola Cluster	140	1.0
Total	**1,468**	**40.4**

1,500-Calorie Menu #5

	Calories	Fiber (g)
Daily allowance: 1 cup skim milk, an orange, and an apple or pear	276	8.2
Breakfast ¾ cup Kellogg's All-Bran with 1 tablespoon raisins and milk from allowance	125	13.3
Light meal 1 cup Libby's canned chili con carne with beans Orange from allowance	276	12.5
Main meal 1 frankfurter Mixed salad: 1 tomato (sliced), a few scallions, 1 cucumber (sliced), chopped lettuce leaves, 1 green pepper (sliced), ½ cup cooked peas (chilled), ½ cup cooked corn (chilled), and 2 tablespoons oil-free French dressing 1 whole-wheat matzo ½ cup fruit-flavored low-fat yogurt	610	19.0
Snacks and drinks Apple or pear from allowance 1 Fibermed biscuit, spread with 1 triangle Laughing Cow cheese and topped with a few cucumber slices 1 drink chosen from chart (page 266) to the value of 100 calories	242	5.7
Total	**1,529**	**58.7**

1,500-Calorie Menu #6

	Calories	Fiber (g)
Daily allowance: 1 cup skim milk, an orange, and an apple or pear	276	8.2
Breakfast ¾ cup Kellogg's All-Bran with 1 tablespoon chopped dried apricots and milk from allowance	126	14.6
Light meal Ham and cheese sandwich: 2 slices of whole-wheat bread filled with 2 tablespoons Oscar Mayer Ham and Cheese Spread and 1 sliced large tomato 1 small (¾-ounce) package of potato chips Apple or pear from allowance	338	5.0
Main meal 1 (12-ounce) package of Green Giant Salisbury Steak with Gravy ½ cup prepared instant mashed potatoes (no butter) ¾ cup frozen mixed vegetables 1 cup fresh blueberries topped with 1 tablespoon Kellogg's Cracklin' Bran	525	18.7
Snacks and drinks Orange from allowance 1 Nature Valley Coconut Granola Bar Drinks chosen from chart (page 266) to the value of 150 calories	271	1.0
Total	**1,536**	**47.5**

Drinking on the F-Plan

Although most men could achieve a very successful weight loss on any of the 1,500-calorie menus in this book, these menus have been especially designed to take into account their different life-styles. The menus, which total between approximately 1,200 and 1,300 calories, are also intended for the drinking person, allowing him or her to "spend" between 200 and 300 calories (to bring the daily total up to 1,500 calories) on alcoholic drinks (see chart, page 266). Those menus with meals eaten in a restaurant, etc., have an *approximate* calorie and fiber total, since it is impossible to calculate the value of such meals accurately.

Varied eating habits have been taken into account in these menus. Although breakfasts have been included each day, if you are a nonbreakfast-eater you can keep this meal until later in the day. Various types of lunches—for example, packed lunches, café, restaurant, business, and Sunday/weekend lunches—have been included to cater to different needs. Some of the evening meals are easy-to-cook meals; others are more elaborate. The recipes are all planned to serve one person, but the recipe ingredients can easily be multiplied by the number of people eating together, when appropriate.

Some variation from the basic F-Plan rules will be found in the daily allowances since some people lack the time to make Fiber-Filler and others find skim milk unacceptable. In case anyone should be tempted to give up the diet for either of these reasons, half the menus do not include Fiber-Filler and a few menus include whole milk (in place of skim milk) in the daily allowance.

Special Diet Notes

1. Decide whether you wish to include one or two alcoholic drinks in your daily menus.

2. Choose a 1,500-calorie menu on days when you can do without alcohol.

3. Choose a 1,200–1,300-calorie menu on days when you know you will want an alcoholic drink, and decide which drinks you will have using the chart (page 266).

4. Make sure that you "spend" only an additional 200 to 300 calories on drinks if you want to achieve good weight loss.

5. Select menus for at least two or three days, preferably one week, at a time, so that you can plan to have the right foods ready at the right time.

6. Don't just choose one menu and repeat it every day. Use a variety of menus, which will ensure a variety of foods and hence a variety of nutrients, which is essential for good health.

7. The daily allowance of essential basic F-Plan diet foods varies throughout the menus. Be sure that you know what is included in the daily allowance of each menu you select.

8. Nonalcoholic drinks, such as sugarless tea and coffee, either black or with skim or whole milk from the daily allowance, "low-calorie"-labeled bottled and canned drinks, and water can be drunk in unlimited amounts at any time of the day.

1,500-Calorie Menu #1
(no additional alcohol)

	Calories	Fiber (g)
Daily allowance: Fiber-Filler, 1 cup skim milk, an orange, and an apple or pear	450	23.0

Breakfast
Fiber-Filler with milk from allowance

Lunch (to carry to work)
* Ham Double-Decker Sandwich
1 small (¾-ounce) package of potato
   chips
Apple or pear from allowance   509   7.2

Evening meal
1 chicken leg and thigh, broiled and skin
   removed
1 large baked potato (page 20) served
   with 1 teaspoon diet margarine
12 Brussels sprouts, cooked
¾ cup carrots, cooked
¼ cup vanilla ice cream with 2 vanilla
   wafers
Orange from allowance   560   10.5

                      Total   **1,519**   **40.7**

* HAM DOUBLE-DECKER SANDWICH   *Serves 1*

3   slices of Pepperidge Farm whole-wheat bread
     Prepared mustard
2   (1-ounce) slices of lean boiled ham
     Chopped lettuce
1   teaspoon diet margarine
1   medium tomato, sliced
1   cucumber, sliced
     Salt and pepper to taste

Spread one slice of bread with mustard and top with a slice of
boiled ham and some lettuce. Spread the second slice of bread
lightly with half the margarine and place spread side up on the
ham. Cover with tomato and cucumber slices and lettuce
leaves. Season with salt and pepper. Spread the third slice of
bread with the remaining margarine, top with second slice of
ham, and place on top of sandwich. Wrap.

1,500-Calorie Menu #2
(*no additional alcohol*)

	Calories	Fiber (g)
Daily allowance: Fiber-Filler, 1 cup whole milk, an orange, and an apple or pear	480	23.0
Breakfast Fiber-Filler with milk from allowance Orange from allowance		
Lunch (to carry to work) *Crunchy Cheese and Tomato Rolls 1 Fibermed Apple/Currant Biscuit Apple or pear from allowance	465	14.0
Evening meal 6 ounces cod or haddock brushed with 1 teaspoon oil and broiled (serve with a wedge of lemon) ¾ cup frozen peas, cooked ½ cup canned tomatoes 1 medium boiled potato (no butter) 1 large juice-packed pineapple ring ¼ cup vanilla ice cream	599	12.2
Total	**1,544**	**49.2**

*CRUNCHY CHEESE AND TOMATO ROLLS   *Serves 1*

2   whole-wheat rolls
2   tablespoons grated Cheddar cheese
2   tablespoons diet mayonnaise

1   large celery stalk, finely chopped
1   medium carrot, grated
2   medium tomatoes, sliced

Split the rolls. Mix the grated cheese with the mayonnaise, celery, and carrot. Spread half the mixture on the bottom half of each roll. Cover with sliced tomato and replace the top half. Wrap.

1,500-Calorie Menu #3
(no additional alcohol)

	Calories	Fiber (g)
Daily allowance: Fiber-Filler, 1 cup whole milk, an orange, and an apple or pear	480	23.0
Breakfast Fiber-Filler with milk from allowance		
Lunch (to carry to work) *Sardine and Celery Sandwiches Apple or pear from allowance	572	6.4
Evening meal 1 (8-ounce) Morton Beef Pie ¾ cup cabbage, cooked ¾ cup carrots, cooked 2 RyKrisp crackers 2 celery stalks Orange from allowance	426	8.5
Total	**1,478**	**37.9**

*SARDINE AND CELERY SANDWICHES   *Serves 1*

4   slices of Pepperidge Farm whole-wheat bread
2   teaspoons diet margarine
2   Underwood sardines in tomato sauce
½   teaspoon vinegar
2   large celery stalks, finely chopped
     Chopped lettuce

Spread the bread with margarine. Mash the sardines with the vinegar and mix with the chopped celery. Spread the sardine filling over two slices of bread. Cover with chopped lettuce and top with the remaining slices of bread. Wrap.

1,500-Calorie Menu #4
(no additional alcohol)

	Calories	Fiber (g)
Daily allowance: Fiber-Filler, 1 cup skim milk, an orange, and an apple or pear	450	23.0
Breakfast Fiber-Filler with milk from allowance		
Business/restaurant lunch or evening meal ½ cantaloupe 6 ounces lean porterhouse steak, broiled 1 baked potato, with 1 teaspoon butter Green or mixed salad without dressing 1 (4-ounce) glass of dry red wine	approx. 833	11.8
Light meal 1 (9½-ounce) can of Campbell's Chunky Split Pea & Ham Soup		

4 wheat crackers (Wheat Thins)		
Orange and apple or pear from allowance	215	8.7
Total	**1,498**	**43.5**

1,500-Calorie Menu #5
(no additional alcohol)

	Calories	Fiber (g)
Daily allowance: Fiber-Filler, 1 cup skim milk, an orange, and an apple or pear	450	23.0
Breakfast Fiber-Filler with milk from allowance		
Café/restaurant lunch Mushroom omelet and ¾ cup french fries		
Apple or pear from allowance (Note: If fresh fruit is not served, omit the dessert and eat the fruit at home later.)	approx. 606	4.4
Evening meal *Kidney Bean, Cauliflower, and Corned Beef Salad		
2 RyKrisp crackers with 2 tablespoons cream cheese		
2 celery stalks		
Orange from allowance	508	19.1
Total	**1,564**	**46.5**

*KIDNEY BEAN, CAULIFLOWER, AND CORNED BEEF SALAD   Serves 1

⅓   cup canned kidney beans, drained
1   cup cauliflower florets
1   small onion, sliced
3   (1-ounce) slices of corned beef, diced
1   green pepper, chopped
2   tablespoons oil-free French dressing
     Dash of curry powder
     Chopped lettuce
1   large tomato, cut into wedges

Put all ingredients in a bowl and toss until well mixed. Let stand for 30 minutes before serving.

1,500-Calorie Menu #6
(no additional alcohol)

	Calories	Fiber (g)
Daily allowance: 1 cup skim milk, an orange, and an apple or pear	276	8.2
Breakfast ¾ cup Kellogg's All-Bran with 1 tablespoon raisins and milk from allowance 1 slice of whole-wheat bread spread with 1 teaspoon diet margarine and 1 teaspoon honey or marmalade	206	14.5
Lunch (to carry to work) *Shrimp and Salad Double-Decker Sandwiches 2 graham crackers Apple or pear from allowance	467	8.6

Evening meal
5 ounces lean pork chop, broiled, with
   fat cut off
2 tablespoons applesauce
½ cup canned mushrooms
¾ cup frozen mixed vegetables
½ cup boiled red-skinned potatoes (no
   butter)
1 RyKrisp cracker
1 celery stalk

Orange from allowance	593	14.7
Total	**1,542**	**46.0**

*SHRIMP AND SALAD DOUBLE-DECKER SANDWICHES   *Serves 1*

3   slices of whole-wheat bread
1   tablespoon diet mayonnaise
4   ounces canned shrimps
1   medium tomato, sliced
1   cucumber, sliced
    Chopped lettuce

Spread all three slices of bread on one side with half the mayonnaise. Mix the shrimps with the remaining mayonnaise and spread on one slice of the bread. Place the second slice of bread on top of the shrimps and cover with the tomato, cucumber, and lettuce. Place the final slice of bread, spread side down, on top of the sandwich. Wrap.

1,500-Calorie Menu #7
(no additional alcohol)

	Calories	Fiber (g)
Daily allowance: 1 cup skim milk, an orange, and an apple or pear	276	8.2
Breakfast		
¾ cup Kellogg's All-Bran with milk from allowance		
1 medium banana	181	15.3
Lunch (to carry to work)		
Cheese and pickle bagel: 1 whole-wheat bagel, split and filled with 2 tablespoons sweet pickle relish mixed with 2 tablespoons grated Cheddar cheese		
1 large carrot, cut into sticks		
1 large celery stalk		
1 small (1-ounce) bag of peanuts		
Orange from allowance	469	8.2
Evening meal		
*Bacon and Liver Casserole		
1 large baked potato (baked in the oven with the casserole—see page 20)		
½ cup canned tomatoes		
¾ cup frozen peas, boiled		
Apple or pear from allowance	604	14.2
Total	**1,530**	**45.9**

*BACON AND LIVER CASSEROLE   *Serves 1*

1   tablespoon cornstarch
⅛   teaspoon basil
     Salt and pepper to taste
¼   pound chicken livers, sliced
2   slices of bacon
1   small onion, sliced
½   beef bouillon cube

Preheat the oven to 350° F. Mix the cornstarch with the basil
and a little salt and pepper. Toss the liver in the mixture. Cut
bacon slices into three pieces. Arrange half the bacon pieces in
an ovenproof dish. Cover with half the onion slices, the liver,
the rest of the onion slices, and finally the remaining bacon
pieces. Dissolve the bouillon cube in ⅓ cup boiling water and
pour over the ingredients in the dish. Cover with a tightly fit-
ting lid or foil and bake in the oven for 1 hour.

1,500-Calorie Menu #8
(no additional alcohol)

	Calories	Fiber (g)
Daily allowance: 1 cup skim milk, an orange, and an apple or pear	276	8.2
Breakfast ⅔ cup Kellogg's All-Bran with milk from allowance	96	12.6
Restaurant/lunch Spaghetti Bolognese Ice cream	approx. 575	1.5

Evening meal
*Fish Bake
1 cup boiled potatoes (no butter)
¾ cup frozen peas, boiled
1 RyKrisp cracker
2 tablespoons cream cheese
2 celery stalks
Orange and apple or pear from
    allowance   601   13.0

                              Total   1,548   35.3

*FISH BAKE   *Serves 1*

6   ounces frozen cod or haddock
4   ounces Campbell's Condensed Cream of Mushroom
     Soup
1   tablespoon skim milk from allowance
1   tablespoon finely chopped onion

Put the fish in the bottom of a small ovenproof dish. Combine
the soup, milk, and onion. Pour over the fish steaks and bake
at 375° F for 30 minutes. Serve hot.

*1,500-Calorie Menu #9
(no additional alcohol)*

	Calories	Fiber (g)
Daily allowance: 1 cup skim milk, an orange, and an apple or pear	276	8.2

Breakfast
¾ cup Kellogg's All-Bran with 1
    tablespoon raisins and milk from
    allowance
Orange from allowance   125   13.3

Lunch (to take to work)
*Tuna on a Whole-Wheat Bagel
1 large carrot, cut into sticks
1 medium tomato, cut into wedges
Peanut Butter & Chocolate Chip
    Crunchola Bar
Apple or pear from allowance   577   9.5

Evening meal
1 (11-ounce) package of Lean Cuisine
    Zucchini Lasagna
1 cup frozen mixed vegetables, cooked
1 medium banana, sliced, to top ½ cup
    plain low-fat yogurt sprinkled with 1
    tablespoon bran   484   11.8

| | **Total** | **1,462** | **42.8** |

*TUNA ON A WHOLE-WHEAT BAGEL

1   whole-wheat bagel
½   cup water-packed tuna, drained and flaked
1   tablespoon diet mayonnaise
1   celery stalk, diced
    A few cucumber slices

Cut the bagel in half. Flake the tuna, mix with mayonnaise and celery, and spread on the bottom half of the bagel. Cover with cucumber and top with the remaining half. Wrap.

1,500-Calorie Menu #10
(no additional alcohol)

	Calories	Fiber (g)
Daily allowance: 1 cup skim milk, an orange, and an apple or pear	276	8.2
Breakfast ¾ cup Kellogg's All-Bran with milk from allowance	96	12.6
Sunday lunch 1 package of Green Giant Swiss Steak in Gravy with Stuffed Potato 12 Brussels sprouts, cooked ¾ cup carrots, boiled *Banana Melba	607	9.1
Evening meal 1 slice of Celeste's Frozen Pizza *Coleslaw 1 Fibermed Apple/Currant Biscuit Orange and apple or pear from allowance	479	12.0
Total	**1,458**	**41.9**

*BANANA MELBA　*Serves 1*

¼　cup frozen vanilla yogurt
½　banana
1　tablespoon raspberry preserves
1　tablespoon orange juice

Spread yogurt on an oval flat dish. Peel the banana, cut it in half, and arrange the halves on either side of the yogurt. Mix the preserves with orange juice and spoon over to serve.

*COLESLAW   *Serves 1*

1   cup shredded white cabbage
⅔   cup grated carrot
1   small onion, finely chopped
1   large celery stalk
2   walnut halves, chopped
2   tablespoons diet mayonnaise

Mix all ingredients thoroughly.

For the Drinking Person #1
1,200–1,300-Calorie Menu

	Calories	Fiber (g)
Daily allowance: Fiber-Filler, 1 cup skim milk, an orange, and an apple or pear	450	23.0
Breakfast Fiber-Filler with milk from allowance		
Lunch (to carry to work) *Liverwurst and Beet Double-Decker Sandwich 1 Fibermed Apple/Currant Biscuit Apple or pear from allowance	409	9.8

Evening meal
*Continental Tuna Stir-Fry
*Strawberry Delight

Orange from allowance	360	6.7
Total	**1,219**	**39.5**

*LIVERWURST AND BEET DOUBLE-DECKER
SANDWICH   *Serves 1*

3   slices of Pepperidge Farm whole-wheat bread
2   teaspoons mustard
2   tablespoons Underwood Liverwurst Spread
     Chopped lettuce
¼   cup sliced pickled beets

Cover a slice of bread with liverwurst spread, mustard, and
lettuce. Top with the second slice of bread. Spread mustard on
the upper surface of the second slice of bread and on one side
of the third slice of bread. Cover the second slice of bread with
beets and lettuce. Place the third slice of bread on top, spread
side down. Wrap.

*CONTINENTAL TUNA STIR-FRY   *Serves 1*

1   cup Birds Eye Chinese Stir-Fry Vegetables
½   cup water-packed tuna, drained

Cook the vegetables according to package directions. Flake
the tuna, stir into the vegetables, and heat through. Put on a
warm serving dish and serve at once.

*STRAWBERRY DELIGHT   *Serves 1*

½   cup low-fat yogurt
1   cup sliced fresh strawberries
3   tablespoons Kellogg's Cracklin' Bran

Top yogurt with strawberries. Sprinkle with cereal.

For the Drinking Person #2
1,200–1,300-Calorie Menu

	Calories	Fiber (g)
Daily allowance: Fiber-Filler, 1 cup skim milk, an orange, and an apple or pear	450	23.0
Breakfast Fiber-Filler with milk from allowance 1 medium banana	85	2.7
Lunch (to carry to work) *Cottage Cheese and Celery Sandwiches Apple or pear from allowance	360	12.4
Evening meal 1 (12¾-ounce) package of Lean Cuisine Chicken and Vegetables with Vermicelli Salad: 1 cucumber (sliced), 2 medium tomatoes (sliced), and 1 large celery stalk (diced) with 1 tablespoon oil-free French dressing and a few chopped chives (optional) Orange from allowance	337	2.3
Total	**1,232**	**40.4**

*COTTAGE CHEESE AND CELERY SANDWICHES   *Serves 1*

½   cup low-fat cottage cheese with chives
1   large celery stalk, finely chopped
¼   cup kidney beans
     Salt and pepper to taste
3   slices of Pepperidge Farm whole-wheat bread
     Chopped lettuce

Mix the cottage cheese with the celery, beans, and salt and pepper. Spread a slice of bread with half of the cottage cheese mixture; top with lettuce, then the second slice of bread, and repeat; top with third slice. Cut into halves or quarters. Wrap.

For the Drinking Person #3
1,200–1,300-Calorie Menu

	Calories	Fiber (g)
Daily allowance: Fiber-Filler, 1 cup skim milk, an orange, and an apple or pear	450	23.0
Breakfast Fiber-Filler with milk from allowance 1 RyKrisp cracker spread with 1 teaspoon diet margarine and 1 teaspoon honey	61	0.9
Business/restaurant lunch or evening meal 6 ounces broiled steak Green or mixed salad without dressing Fresh fruit approx.	520	7.0

Light meal
Baked beans on toast: 1 slice of Arnold
   whole-wheat bread, toasted, ⅔ cup
   canned baked beans in tomato sauce,
   and 1 egg, poached
Orange and apple or pear from
   allowance

	333	17.8
Total approx. 1,364		**48.7**

For the Drinking Person #4
1,200–1,300-Calorie Menu

	Calories	Fiber (g)
Daily allowance: Fiber-Filler, 1 cup skim milk, an orange, and an apple or pear	450	23.0
Breakfast Fiber-Filler with milk from allowance		
Deli sandwich lunch 1 ham sandwich on a whole-wheat bread or roll ½ cup pickled bean salad approx.	515	8.0
Evening meal *Chicken Salad *Prune Compote	383	18.4
Total	**1,348**	**49.4**

*CHICKEN SALAD   *Serves 1*

½   cup cooked diced chicken
1   cup shredded red or white cabbage
1   teaspoon finely chopped onion
1   apple (from allowance), cored and chopped
2   teaspoons lemon juice
2   tablespoons oil-free French dressing
     Salt and pepper to taste
     A few leaves lettuce
     A few parsley sprigs
     A few cucumber slices

Remove any skin from chicken and dice meat. Put the cabbage, onion, and apple in a bowl. Add the lemon juice and French dressing and mix well. Season with salt and pepper. Arrange the cabbage salad on a serving dish with the diced chicken, lettuce, parsley, and cucumber.

*PRUNE COMPOTE   *Serves 1*

4   dried prunes
4   drops angostura bitters (optional)
     Strip of lemon peel
1   teaspoon sugar
1   orange (from allowance), sectioned
½   banana, peeled and sliced

Cover the prunes with cold water and leave overnight. Put the prunes and liquid in a pan and add the bitters and lemon peel. Cover and simmer for 20 minutes. Remove the lemon peel and stir in the sugar. If serving hot, add the orange segments and sliced banana, heat through, and serve. If serving cold, let the prunes cool before adding the orange and banana.

For the Drinking Person #5
1,200–1,300-Calorie Menu

	Calories	Fiber (g)
Daily allowance: Fiber-Filler, 1 cup skim milk, an orange, and an apple or pear	450	23.0
Breakfast Fiber-Filler with milk from allowance		
Lunch (to carry to work or eat at home) 1 cup Progresso Lentil Soup 4 RyKrisp crackers spread with ¼ cup Cheddar cheese Apple or pear from allowance	364	6.8
Evening meal *Mixed Vegetable Curry with Rice Orange from allowance	430	28.3
Total	**1,244**	**58.1**

*MIXED VEGETABLE CURRY WITH RICE   *Serves 1*

½   cup brown rice
1   tablespoon diet margarine
1   small onion, chopped
¼   small apple, cored and chopped
½   teaspoon curry powder
1   teaspoon flour
½   cup vegetable stock or water
1   teaspoon tomato purée
1   teaspoon lemon juice
½   cup canned kidney beans
¾   cup frozen mixed vegetables

¼   cup fresh mushrooms, sliced
     Salt and pepper to taste

Boil the rice in lightly salted water for about 25 minutes, or until tender. While the rice is cooking, melt the margarine in a saucepan. Add the onion and apple and cook gently for 5 minutes. Stir in the curry powder and flour. Add the stock, bring to a boil, stirring, then add the tomato purée and lemon juice. Cover and simmer for 5 minutes. Add the kidney beans, mixed vegetables, and mushrooms. Bring to a boil, cover, and simmer gently for 15 minutes. Season with salt and pepper. Drain the rice and serve with the vegetable curry.

For the Drinking Person #6
1,200–1,300-Calorie Menu

	Calories	Fiber (g)
Daily allowance: 1 cup skim milk, an orange, and an apple or pear	276	8.2
Breakfast ¾ cup Kellogg's All-Bran and milk from allowance	96	12.6
Restaurant/café lunch Tomato soup (or any other soup you wish) Chicken salad (no salad dressing)	approx. 385	3.0
Evening meal *Cheese and Spinach Omelet ½ cup canned baked beans in tomato sauce *Fruit Salad	517	25.5
Total approx.	**1,274**	**49.3**

*CHEESE AND SPINACH OMELET   *Serves 1*

2   eggs
1   cup frozen chopped spinach, thawed
    Salt and pepper to taste
1   teaspoon diet margarine
¼   cup grated Cheddar cheese

Lightly beat the eggs with 2 tablespoons water. Stir in the thawed spinach and salt and pepper. Grease a nonstick omelet pan or small frying pan with margarine and heat the pan. Pour in the egg and spinach mixture and heat until set. Sprinkle the grated cheese over the omelet and continue to heat for 1 minute. Fold the omelet in half and turn out onto a warm plate. Serve at once.

*FRUIT SALAD   *Serves 1*

1   orange (from allowance), sectioned
1   apple or pear (from allowance), cored and diced or sliced
10 black grapes, halved and seeded
¼   cup diet ginger ale
1   teaspoon slivered almonds

Mix the orange sections, apple or pear, and grapes with the ginger ale. Sprinkle on the slivered almonds and serve immediately.

For the Drinking Person #7
1,200–1,300-Calorie Menu

	Calories	Fiber (g)
Daily allowance: 1 cup skim milk, an orange, and an apple or pear	276	8.2

Breakfast
1⅓ cups Kellogg's 40% Bran Flakes
    with milk from allowance   141   7.8

Lunch (to carry to work)
Peanut butter and fig sandwich: 2 slices
    of Arnold whole-wheat bread, 1
    tablespoon peanut butter, and 2
    tablespoons chopped figs
1 carrot, cut into sticks
1 large celery stalk
Apple or pear from allowance   302   11.0

Evening meal
*Beef in Red Wine Sauce
1 cup broccoli, cooked
1 Fibermed Apple/Currant Biscuit
Orange from allowance   526   23.2

Total	**1,245**	**50.2**

*BEEF IN RED WINE SAUCE   *Serves 1*

¼   pound lean flank steak, sliced
½   cup cannellini beans, drained
½   cup canned Franco-American Beef Gravy
1   tablespoon red wine

Arrange the flank steak slices in an ovenproof dish. Spoon the beans over the steak. Combine gravy and wine and spoon over. Cover and bake in the oven at 350°F for 1 hour.

For the Drinking Person #8
1,200–1,300-Calorie Menu

	Calories	Fiber (g)
Daily allowance: 1 cup skim milk, an orange, and an apple or pear	276	8.2
Breakfast ½ cup Kellogg's All-Bran with 1 medium banana (sliced) and milk from allowance	106	9.8
Lunch (to take to work) Bologna with bagel: Cut a whole-wheat bagel and spread the cut surfaces with 1 tablespoon sweet pickle plus 1 teaspoon prepared mustard. Top with two slices of Oscar Mayer bologna. 1 small tomato, sliced 1 large celery stalk, cut into short sticks Orange from allowance	387	5.0
Evening meal 1 (5-ounce) lean loin lamb chop, broiled 2 teaspoons mint jelly ½ cup canned lima beans, cooked ½ cup canned tomatoes, heated ½ cup boiled potatoes (no butter) Apple or pear from allowance	551	14.1
Total	**1,320**	**37.1**

For the Drinking Person #9
1,200–1,300-Calorie Menu

	Calories	Fiber (g)
Daily allowance: 1 cup whole milk, an orange, and an apple or pear	335	8.2
Breakfast ¾ cup Kellogg's All-Bran with milk from allowance	96	12.6
Restaurant lunch Grilled Dover sole Mixed salad without dressing Fruit sherbet approx.	620	2.0
Evening meal Baked beans on toast: 1 slice of Arnold whole-wheat bread, toasted, topped with ⅔ cup canned baked beans in tomato sauce, heated Orange and apple or pear from allowance	255	17.8
Total	**1,306**	**40.6**

For the Drinking Person #10
1,200–1,300-Calorie Menu

	Calories	Fiber (g)
Daily allowance: 1 cup whole milk, an orange, and an apple or pear	335	8.2
Breakfast		
¾ cup Kellogg's All-Bran and 1 tablespoon raisins and milk from allowance	125	13.4
Sunday/weekend lunch		
½ chicken breast, roasted, and skin removed		
1 large baked potato (page 20), served with 1 teaspoon diet margarine		
⅔ cup canned corn		
¼ cup button mushrooms		
½ cup juice-packed pear halves over ½ cup plain low-fat yogurt	510	13.4
Evening meal		
*Egg Salad		
1 slice of Arnold whole-wheat bread spread with 1 teaspoon diet margarine		
Orange and apple or pear from allowance	308	7.3
Total	**1,278**	**42.3**

*EGG SALAD   *Serves 1*

1   egg, hard-boiled
¼   cup diced canned mushrooms
1   tablespoon lemon juice
     Salt and pepper to taste
     A few lettuce leaves
1   tomato, sliced
⅔   cup carrot, grated
2   tablespoons diced pickled beets
¼   cup green pepper
1   tablespoon diet mayonnaise

Shell and halve the egg. Combine mushrooms and lemon juice. Season with salt and pepper. Arrange a bed of lettuce on a plate, then arrange the halved egg, mushrooms, sliced tomato, grated carrot, beets, and green pepper on top. Pour the salad dressing over the egg.

F-Plan for Children

Most children will hardly know they are on a diet when following these menus, since the F-Plan allows children to eat the foods they like.

Although most diets that allow a daily intake of 1,500 calories are quite safe for school-age children to follow, they are rarely planned with children in mind and hence do not include their favorite foods.

A daily calorie allowance of 1,500 will achieve a good weight loss for most boys; the weight loss for girls (unless very overweight) may be less spectacular. So long as there is no further weight gain or, better still, if there is a steady (even if small) weight loss, then they will have a chance to "grow into their weight."

The following menus follow the basic F-Plan diet rules, and include those foods that my testers and junior informers tell me are most popular with children. All the daily menus provide approximately 1,500 calories and between 35 g and 0 g of fiber.

The first ten menus include a daily portion of Fiber-Filler (page 13) in the daily allowance; however, since some children do not like Fiber-Filler and would find a diet including it every day quite unacceptable, there are ten daily menus without Fiber-Filler. These all contain a bran-based breakfast cereal, which partly replaces the Fiber-Filler. Also in the daily allowance, all twenty menus include two whole pieces of fruit (an orange and an apple or pear) and 2 cups of skim milk. The quantity of milk has been increased from the basic F-Plan diet allowance to ensure that children obtain adequate amounts of nutrients for their growth requirements.

Special Diet Notes

1. Choose a week's menus at one time so that the food can be bought in advance.

2. Don't swap meals from one day's menu to another. Stick to the chosen menus—there should be sufficient to choose from for you to avoid foods which your children particularly dislike. However, the same menu every day will not provide you with sufficient variety of foods and will be very boring. You do need to use several menus if your children are dieting for more than a few days.

3. The skim milk allowance is used on the breakfast cereal or Fiber-Filler.

4. Your kids can drink canned and bottled drinks labeled "diet" and as much water as they like throughout the day.

5. The daily menus are divided up into breakfast, midmorning snack, lunch, after-school snack, dinner, and a bedtime drink or snack. However, if this meal plan does not fit in with your life-style then you can rearrange the meals (for example, eat the evening meal at lunchtime and keep the midmorning snack until lunchtime or the evening) so long as at the end of the day your children have eaten only those foods on the daily menu.

6. Some of the lunches are suitable for packing, so they can be eaten at school or on a picnic. Soups and salads can be packed as well as sandwiches—just remember to send the right tools along to eat them with.

7. The after-school snack becomes a midafternoon snack on weekends.

8. Finally, your children should eat more slowly than they usually do. Foods high in fiber need more chewing than low-fiber foods, so they will probably slow down anyway. Slow eating means that they have time to enjoy their food and should feel more satisfied at the end of a meal, whereas if they gobble their food down they forget all too quickly that they have eaten and want more food.

9. Remember that if your children stick to their diet, not only will they be more fit and healthier, but life will be more fun.

1,500-Calorie Menu #1 with Fiber-Filler

	Calories	Fiber (g)
Daily allowance: Fiber-Filler, 2 cups skim milk, an orange, and an apple or pear	511	23.0
Breakfast Half portion of Fiber-Filler with milk from allowance Orange from allowance		
Midmorning snack 1 Nature Valley Oats and Honey Granola Bar	150	1.0
Lunch *Peanut Butter and Jelly Sandwich 1 medium carrot, cut into sticks 1 cucumber, sliced Apple or pear from allowance	338	7.0
After-school snack Remaining Fiber-Filler with milk from allowance		
Evening meal 4 ounces hamburger, broiled ½ cup canned baked beans in tomato sauce 1 medium potato, boiled and mashed ¼ cup vanilla ice cream	434	14.5
Bedtime drink A cup of chocolate: 1 tablespoon Hershey's chocolate syrup with milk from allowance	53	0.0
Total	**1,486**	**45.5**

*PEANUT BUTTER AND JELLY SANDWICH

2   slices of Arnold whole-wheat bread
2   tablespoons peanut butter
1   tablespoon Featherweight Low-Calorie Strawberry
     Preserves

Spread one slice of bread with the peanut butter and the other
with jelly. Combine slices. Wrap.

1,500-Calorie Menu #2 with Fiber-Filler

	Calories	Fiber (g)
Daily allowance: Fiber-Filler with 2 cups skim milk, an orange, and an apple or pear	511	23.0
Breakfast Half portion of Fiber-Filler with milk from allowance 1 slice of Pepperidge Farm whole-wheat bread, toasted and spread with 1 teaspoon diet margarine	81	1.2
Midmorning snack 2 graham crackers	54	1.4
Lunch 2 large brown-and-serve pork sausages, broiled 1 RyKrisp cracker 2 medium tomatoes, sliced 1 large celery stalk, cut into short lengths Apple or pear from allowance	286	2.7

After-school snack
Remaining Fiber-Filler with skim milk
  from allowance
Orange from allowance

Evening meal
*Pasta with Meat Sauce
1 medium banana   489   8.8

Bedtime drink
A cup of chocolate: 1 tablespoon
  Hershey's chocolate syrup with milk
  from allowance   53   0.0
                                          ─────────────────────
                        Total   **1,474**   **37.1**

*PASTA WITH MEAT SAUCE   *Serves 1*
(Several portions of meat sauce can be made up at one time
and frozen until required.)

¾   cup whole-wheat spaghetti

MEAT SAUCE
¼   pound ground beef
1   small onion, peeled and finely chopped
1   celery stalk, finely diced
¼   beef bouillon cube, dissolved in ⅓ cup boiling water
    Salt and pepper to taste
    A pinch of basil and oregano
1   teaspoon tomato purée
¼   cup canned baked beans in tomato sauce

Fry the ground beef in a nonstick saucepan until well browned. Drain off all the fat that has cooked out of the meat. Add the onion, celery, and bouillon to the meat in the pan and bring to a boil, stirring. Reduce the heat, season with salt and pepper, and add herbs and tomato purée. Cover and simmer gently for 30 minutes, stirring occasionally and adding more water if necessary to prevent the mixture from sticking. Boil the pasta in salted water for about 12 minutes, or until just tender. Drain and arrange on a plate. Stir the baked beans into the meat sauce and heat through for 2 to 3 minutes, then spoon over the pasta.

1,500-Calorie Menu #3 with Fiber-Filler

	Calories	Fiber (g)
Daily allowance: Fiber-Filler, 2 cups skim milk, an orange, and an apple or pear	511	23.0
Breakfast Half portion of Fiber-Filler with milk from allowance 1 egg, boiled 1 slice of Arnold whole-wheat bread, spread with 1 teaspoon diet jelly	149	1.2
Midmorning snack Apple or pear from allowance		
Lunch *Ham and Cheese Rolls *Corny Coleslaw Orange from allowance	307	5.5

After-school snack
Remaining Fiber-Filler with skim milk
   from allowance

Evening meal		
2 fish sticks, baked		
¾ cup frozen peas, cooked		
½ cup frozen french fries, baked		
½ cup fruit-flavored yogurt	493	12.6

Bedtime drink		
A cup of chocolate: 1 tablespoon		
Hershey's chocolate syrup with milk		
from allowance	53	0.0
Total	**1,513**	**42.3**

HAM AND CHEESE ROLLS   *Serves 1*

¼   cup cottage cheese with pineapple
1   celery stalk, diced
2   thin slices of lean boiled ham

Mix the cottage cheese with celery. Divide equally between
the two slices of ham and spread over the ham. Roll up the
ham and secure with a toothpick.

CORNY COLESLAW   *Serves 1*

½   cup shredded white cabbage
⅔   cup grated carrot
⅓   cup canned corn, drained
1   tablespoon diet mayonnaise

Mix together the cabbage, carrot, and corn. Stir in the salad
dressing.

1,500-Calorie Menu #4 with Fiber-Filler

	Calories	Fiber (g)
Daily allowance: Fiber-Filler, 2 cups skim milk, an orange, and an apple or pear	511	23.0
Breakfast Half portion of Fiber-Filler with milk from allowance 1 medium banana	85	2.7
Midmorning snack 1 Nature Valley Honey 'N Oats Granola Bar	150	1.0
Lunch *Cheese and Bean Bagel 1 raw carrot, cut into sticks Apple or pear from allowance	332	11.3
After-school snack 1½ tablespoons Planter's Soy Nuts	95	1.0
Evening meal 2 chicken drumsticks, broiled, skin removed ⅓ cup canned corn ¼ cup canned mushrooms 2 medium tomatoes 1 cup skim milk from allowance mixed with 1½ teaspoons Hershey's chocolate syrup	339	5.0
Bedtime snack Orange from allowance		
Total	**1,512**	**44.0**

*CHEESE AND BEAN BAGEL   *Serves 1*

1   whole-wheat bagel
2   tablespoons grated Cheddar cheese
¼   cup canned baked beans in tomato sauce
     Pepper to taste
     Dash of Worcestershire sauce (optional)
     Chopped lettuce

Split the bagel in half lengthwise. Mash the grated cheese and beans together, using a fork. Season with pepper and add Worcestershire sauce. Spread the cheese and bean mixture on the bottom half of the bagel. Top with chopped lettuce and the other half of the bagel.

1,500-Calorie Menu #5 with Fiber-Filler

	Calories	Fiber (g)
Daily allowance: Fiber-Filler, 2 cups skim milk, an orange, and an apple or pear	511	23.0
Breakfast Fiber-Filler with milk from allowance		
Midmorning snack 1 slice of Arnold whole-wheat bread, toasted and spread with 1 teaspoon diet margarine and 2 teaspoons honey	111	1.2
Lunch *Bean and Sausage Soup 2 RyKrisp crackers Apple or pear from allowance	374	26.4

After-school snack
1 graham cracker   27   0.7

Evening meal
1 (5-ounce) lean loin lamb chop, broiled
12 Brussels sprouts or ¾ cup cooked
    cabbage
⅔ cup frozen mixed vegetables, cooked
Orange from allowance   425   9.2

Bedtime drink
A cup of chocolate: 1 tablespoon
    Hershey's chocolate syrup with skim
    milk from allowance   53   0.0

                              Total   1,501   60.5

BEAN AND SAUSAGE SOUP   Serves 1

¾ cup canned baked beans in tomato sauce
⅔ cup grated carrot
1 beef bouillon cube
   Freshly ground pepper to taste
1 brown-and-serve pork sausage

Put the baked beans and grated carrot in a saucepan. Dissolve
the bouillon cube in ½ cup boiling water and stir into the beans
and carrot. Bring to a boil, cover, and simmer gently for 15 to
20 minutes. Meanwhile, panfry the sausage until well done,
then cut it into slices. Add to the soup, taste for seasoning, and
add a little boiling water if the soup is too thick. Serve hot with
RyKrisps.

1,500-Calorie Menu #6 with Fiber-Filler

	Calories	Fiber (g)
Daily allowance: Fiber-Filler, 2 cups skim milk, an orange, and an apple or pear	511	23.0
Breakfast Half portion of Fiber-Filler with milk from allowance Orange from allowance		
Midmorning snack 2 tablespoons Planter's Soy Nuts	126	7.2
Lunch *Sardine Sandwich	418	4.5
After-school snack Apple or pear from allowance		
Evening meal *Meaty Baked Potato ½ cup diet gelatin dessert	439	4.6
Bedtime snack Remaining Fiber-Filler with milk from allowance		
Total	**1,494**	**39.3**

*SARDINE SANDWICH   *Serves 1*

2   sardines canned in tomato sauce
2   tablespoons cottage cheese
     Salt and pepper to taste
2   slices of Arnold whole-wheat bread
2   lettuce leaves
     A few slices of cucumber

Mash the sardines with the cottage cheese and season. Fill the two slices of bread with the sardine mixture, lettuce, and cucumber.

*MEATY BAKED POTATO   *Serves 1*

1   large potato
¼   pound ground beef
1   small onion, chopped
¼   cup finely chopped celery
1   teaspoon tomato paste or purée
     Salt and pepper to taste

Scrub the potato well, then bake by one of the methods described on page 20. Meanwhile, fry the ground beef in a saucepan without added fat until well browned. Drain off and discard the fat. Add the onion, celery, tomato paste, and ⅓ cup water. Heat to a boil, then simmer, covered, for 15 minutes. Cut the baked potato in half lengthwise, scoop out some of the flesh, and mix with the hot ground beef mixture. Season. Pile back into the jackets and serve.

1,500-Calorie Menu #7 with Fiber-Filler

	Calories	Fiber (g)
Daily allowance: Fiber-Filler, 2 cups skim milk, an orange, and an apple or pear	511	23.0
Breakfast Half portion of Fiber-Filler with milk from allowance 1 large slice of Pepperidge Farm whole-wheat bread, toasted and spread with 1 teaspoon diet margarine	81	11.2
Midmorning snack Apple or pear from allowance		
Lunch 1 (15-ounce) can of Buitoni Spaghetti with Sauce, sprinkled with 2 tablespoons bran ½ cup canned corn Orange from allowance	408	6.0
After-school snack Remaining Fiber-Filler with milk from allowance		
Evening meal *Hungarian Liver ¾ cup cabbage, boiled	448	6.5
Bedtime drink Mix 2 tablespoons diet orange soda with ½ cup milk from allowance 2 graham crackers	54	1.4
Total	**1,502**	**48.1**

*HUNGARIAN LIVER   *Serves 1*

¼   pound chicken livers
1   tablespoon whole-wheat flour
1   tablespoon diet margarine
1   small onion, thinly sliced
5   mushrooms, sliced
½   cup beef bouillon (made from ½ bouillon cube)
1   teaspoon tomato purée
⅓   cup whole-wheat macaroni
1   tablespoon yogurt

Cut up the livers. Toss in the flour to coat. Heat the margarine
in a nonstick pan and cook the onion over low heat until soft.
Add the mushrooms and cook for 2 to 3 minutes. Add the liver
and cook for 3 minutes. Stir in the bouillon and tomato purée.
Bring to a boil, cover, and simmer gently for 10 minutes.
Meanwhile, cook the macaroni in lightly salted boiling water
for 12 to 15 minutes, until just soft. Drain the macaroni well
and arrange on a serving plate. Spoon the liver mixture on top.
Spoon the yogurt on top of the liver and pasta.

1,500-Calorie Menu #8 with Fiber-Filler

	Calories	Fiber (g)
Daily allowance: Fiber-Filler, 2 cups skim milk, an orange, and an apple or pear	511	23.0
Breakfast Half portion of Fiber-Filler with milk from allowance		
1 slice of whole-wheat bread, spread with 1 slice cheese; broil until cheese melts	154	1.2

Midmorning snack
Apple or pear from allowance

Lunch
*Tuna Salad
1 slice of whole-wheat bread   333   5.8

After-school snack
Remaining Fiber-Filler with milk from
    allowance

Evening meal
*One-Pan Supper
¼ cup vanilla ice cream served with
    orange from allowance, sectioned   445   9.0

Bedtime drink
A cup of chocolate: 1 tablespoon
    Hershey's chocolate syrup with milk
    from allowance   53

Total	**1,494**	**39.0**

*TUNA SALAD   *Serves 1*

½   cup water-packed tuna, drained
¼   cup whole-wheat pasta shells, cooked
½   cup canned corn
1   celery stalk, diced
2   tablespoons low-fat yogurt
    Salt and pepper to taste

Flake the tuna into a bowl. Add the pasta, corn, and celery and
mix well. Add salt and pepper and yogurt and toss gently until
well mixed.

*ONE-PAN SUPPER   *Serves 1*

2	eggs
	Salt and pepper to taste
1	tablespoon diet margarine
1	small chopped onion
1	small cooked potato, diced
1	medium fresh tomato, chopped
5	mushrooms, sliced
1	heaping tablespoon cooked peas

Beat the eggs together with 2 tablespoons water and salt and pepper. Melt the margarine in a nonstick frying pan. Add the onion, potato, tomato, and mushrooms and cook over low heat for 5 minutes, stirring frequently. Add the peas, then pour in the beaten eggs. Cook over moderate heat until the egg mixture is set on the bottom, then place under a hot broiler to set the top and brown slightly. Turn out onto a warm plate and serve immediately.

1,500-Calorie Menu #9 with Fiber-Filler

	Calories	Fiber (g)
Daily allowance: Fiber-Filler, 2 cups skim milk, an orange, and an apple or pear	511	23.0
Breakfast Half portion of Fiber-Filler with milk from allowance		
1 medium banana	85	2.7
Midmorning snack 1 Nature Valley Honey 'N Oats Granola Bar	150	1.0

Lunch
*Soft Dinner Rolls
Chopped lettuce
Apple or pear from allowance   362   4.0

After-school snack
Remaining Fiber-Filler with milk from
    allowance

Evening meal
*Quick Fish Pie
½ cup D-Zerta gelatin with orange from
    allowance, sectioned   382   9.2

Bedtime drink
2 tablespoons diet orange soda mixed
    with ½ cup milk from allowance   0   0.0

Total	**1,490**	**39.9**

SOFT DINNER ROLLS   *Serves 1*

2   slices of whole-wheat bread
2   tablespoons chopped sweet pickle
2   slices Oscar Mayer bologna

Flatten the bread with a rolling pin. Spread each slice with 1
tablespoon sweet pickle. Place a slice of bologna on each slice
of bread, roll the bread, and secure with a toothpick.

QUICK FISH PIE   *Serves 1*

½   package Gorton's Sole with Lemon Butter, cooked
½   cup frozen peas, boiled
½   cup prepared instant mashed potatoes (no butter)
1   tablespoon grated Cheddar cheese

Cook the fish according to package directions. Put the peas in a heatproof dish. Top with fish and sauce. Spoon the potato around the edge of the dish. Top with grated cheese and heat through under the broiler until the cheese has melted and is lightly browned.

1,500-Calorie Menu #10 with Fiber-Filler

	Calories	Fiber (g)
Daily allowance: Fiber-Filler, 2 cups skim milk, an orange, and an apple or pear	511	23.0
Breakfast Half portion of Fiber-Filler with milk from allowance 1 slice of whole-wheat bread, toasted and spread with 1 teaspoon diet margarine	81	1.2
Midmorning snack Apple or pear from allowance		
Lunch *Vegetable and Lentil Soup 2 RyKrisp crackers	256	11.8
After-school snack 1 Nature Valley Honey 'N Oats Granola Bar Orange from allowance	150	1.0
Evening meal *Cheese Omelet ½ cup french fries, baked ⅓ cup peas, cooked	501	5.6

Bedtime snack
Remaining Fiber-Filler with milk from
  allowance

	Total	**1,499**	**42.6**

*VEGETABLE AND LENTIL SOUP   *Serves 1*
(A larger amount can be made up at one time and frozen in
individual portions for future use.)

1   small onion, sliced
1   medium carrot, sliced
1   large celery stalk, chopped
¼   cup uncooked lentils
1   chicken bouillon cube
    Salt and pepper to taste

Put the vegetables in a pot with the lentils. Dissolve the bouillon cube in 1½ cups boiling water. (Vegetarians can omit the
bouillon cube.) Add to the pot, with salt and pepper. Bring to a
boil, cover, and simmer gently for 1 hour.

*CHEESE OMELET   *Serves 1*

2   eggs
1   tablespoon bran
    Salt and pepper to taste
1   teaspoon diet margarine
2   tablespoons grated Cheddar cheese

Beat the eggs with 2 tablespoons water, bran, and salt and
pepper. Melt the margarine in a nonstick omelet pan. Pour in
the egg mixture and cook over a moderate heat until set. Sprinkle the cheese over the surface and allow to melt. Fold the
omelet in half and turn out onto a warm plate. Serve at once.

1,500-Calorie Menu #1 no Fiber-Filler

	Calories	Fiber (g)
Daily allowance: 2 cups skim milk, an orange, and an apple or pear	366	8.2
Breakfast ¾ cup Kellogg's All-Bran with skim milk from allowance	96	12.6
Midmorning snack Apple or pear from allowance 2 tablespoons raisins	58	1.4
Lunch *Pita Filled with Corned Beef, Beets, and Cucumber Orange from allowance	343	7.7
After-school snack 1 Ry-Krisp cracker spread with ½ triangle Laughing Cow cheese	37	0.9
Evening meal 2 ounces ham steak, broiled 1 tablespoon prepared mustard 1 large potato, baked (page 20) ½ cup canned lima beans *Stewed Blueberries and Apple Crème	551	20.4
Bedtime drink A cup of chocolate: 1 tablespoon Hershey's chocolate syrup with milk from allowance	53	0.0
Total	**1,504**	**51.2**

*PITA FILLED WITH CORNED BEEF, BEETS, AND CUCUMBER   *Serves 1*

1   large whole-wheat pita
2   slices corned beef
2   tablespoons chopped pickled beets
½   cucumber, finely diced
2   tablespoons three-bean salad

Cut the pita in half. Fill with corned beef, beets, cucumber, and bean salad.

*STEWED BLUEBERRIES AND APPLE CRÈME
Serves 1

¼   cup blueberries
1   apple, cored and sliced
1   teaspoon sugar
½   cup plain low-fat yogurt
1   teaspoon bran

Cook the blueberries and apple with 2 tablespoons water in a covered pan until the fruit is tender. Stir in sugar. Let cool. Serve in a dessert dish, topped with yogurt and sprinkled with bran.

1,500-Calorie Menu #2 no Fiber-Filler

	Calories	Fiber (g)
Daily allowance: 2 cups skim milk, an orange, and an apple or pear	366	8.2
Breakfast 1 cup Kellogg's Raisin Bran with milk from allowance 1 medium banana	215	13.0
Midmorning snack 1 RyKrisp cracker spread with 1 teaspoon diet margarine	41	0.9
Lunch *Welsh Soup with Whole-Wheat Croutons Apple or pear from allowance	163	5.0
After-school snack 1 Nature Valley Raisin Granola Cluster	140	1.0
Evening meal *Egg and Beans with Cheese Crumble Topping ¼ cup vanilla ice cream with orange from allowance, sectioned	538	12.5
Bedtime snack and drink 1 RyKrisp cracker and 1 teaspoon diet jelly 2 tablespoons diet orange soda mixed with ½ cup milk from allowance	34	0.9
Total	**1,497**	**41.5**

*WELSH SOUP WITH WHOLE-WHEAT CROUTONS   *Serves 1*

(Several portions can be made up at one time and frozen in individual portions for future use.)

1   large leek, with coarse green leaves trimmed off
1   medium unpeeled potato, thinly sliced or diced
1   tablespoon bran
½   chicken or vegetable bouillon cube
    Salt and pepper to taste
1   slice of whole-wheat bread

Slice the leek and put in a pot with the potato and bran. Dissolve the ½ bouillon cube in 1 cup boiling water and pour into the pot. Season with salt and pepper. Bring to a boil, cover, and simmer gently for 20 minutes. Purée the soup in a blender or food processor. Reheat, check seasoning, and thin with water, if necessary. Toast the bread and cut into small croutons. Serve the soup with the croutons sprinkled on top.

*EGG AND BEANS WITH CHEESE CRUMBLE TOPPING   *Serves 1*

⅓   cup canned baked beans in tomato sauce
1   egg
2   medium tomatoes, sliced
2   tablespoons whole-wheat bread crumbs
1   tablespoon grated Cheddar cheese

Heat the beans and poach the egg. Spoon half the beans into a small ovenproof dish. Place the poached egg on top and then spoon over the remaining beans. Cover with the sliced tomatoes. Mix the bread crumbs with the cheese and sprinkle over the top. Grill until crisp and bubbly.

1,500-Calorie Menu #3 no Fiber-Filler

	Calories	Fiber (g)
Daily allowance: 2 cups skim milk, an orange, and an apple or pear	366	8.2
Breakfast ¾ cup Kellogg's All-Bran with 1 tablespoon raisins and milk from allowance	125	13.3
Midmorning snack Apple or pear from allowance		
Lunch *Cheese with Nutty Coleslaw Orange from allowance	333	11.3
After-school snack 2 graham crackers	54	1.4
Evening meal ½ Stouffer's French Bread Cheese Pizza Green salad: a few lettuce leaves (shredded) 1 cucumber (sliced), 1 green pepper (chopped), and 1 medium tomato (chopped) ½ cup dessert gelatin (any flavor) ¼ cup vanilla ice cream	546	4.7
Bedtime snack 1 RyKrisp cracker spread with ½ triangle Laughing Cow cheese	62	0.9
Total	**1,486**	**39.8**

*CHEESE WITH NUTTY COLESLAW *Serves 1*

1   cup shredded white cabbage
⅔   cup grated carrot
2   tablespoons cooked peas
⅓   cup canned corn
2   tablespoons chopped walnuts
1   tablespoon diet mayonnaise
2   tablespoons grated Swiss cheese (or your favorite)

Mix the vegetables and nuts in a bowl. Stir in the mayonnaise.
Arrange the coleslaw on a plate and pile the grated cheese on
top.

1,500-Calorie Menu #4 no Fiber-Filler

	Calories	Fiber (g)
Daily allowance: 2 cups skim milk, an orange, and an apple or pear	366	8.2
Breakfast 1 cup Kellogg's Raisin Bran with milk from allowance 1 slice of whole-wheat bread spread with 1 teaspoon diet margarine	211	11.5
Midmorning snack Apple or pear from allowance		
Lunch 1 (3-ounce) hamburger, broiled ½ cup canned baked beans in tomato sauce Orange from allowance	290	12.5

After-school snack
1 slice of whole-wheat bread spread with 1 teaspoon diet margarine and 2 teaspoons honey	141	1.2

Evening meal
*Individual Shepherd's Pie
1 cup cabbage, boiled	399	16.3

Bedtime drink
A cup of chocolate: 1 tablespoon Hershey's chocolate syrup with milk from allowance	53	0.0
Total	**1,460**	**49.7**

*INDIVIDUAL SHEPHERD'S PIE   Serves 1

2	ounces ground beef
1	medium onion, finely chopped
⅔	cup grated carrot
½	cup peas, uncooked
¼	cup corn, cooked
1	teaspoon whole-wheat flour
	Salt and pepper to taste
¼	cup beef bouillon (made from ¼ bouillon cube)
1	tablespoon tomato purée
1	teaspoon diet margarine, melted
1	tablespoon bran

Fry the ground beef in a pan until well browned, then drain off and discard fat that has cooked out of the meat. Add the vegetables, flour, and salt and pepper to the meat in the pan. Blend the bouillon with the tomato purée and stir into the meat and vegetables. Heat to a boil, stirring constantly, then cook for 5 minutes, until the mixture thickens. Spoon into a small oven-proof dish. Melt margarine and mix with bran. Sprinkle bran over dish. Bake at 400°F for 30 minutes, or until bubbly.

1,500-Calorie Menu #5 no Fiber-Filler

	Calories	Fiber (g)
Daily allowance: 2 cups skim milk, an orange, and an apple or pear	366	8.2
Breakfast ¾ cup Kellogg's 40% Bran Flakes with milk from allowance 1 egg, poached and served on 1 slice of whole-wheat bread, toasted, no butter	222	6.0
Midmorning snack Orange from allowance		
Lunch *Cottage Cheese and Raisin Sandwich 1 medium carrot, cut into sticks ½ cup fruit-flavored yogurt	400	9.0
After-school snack Apple or pear from allowance		
Evening meal *Macaroni and Vegetable Cheese Bake Green salad: a few lettuce leaves (shredded), a cucumber (chopped), 1 green pepper (chopped), a few sprigs of parsley, and 1 tomato (sliced) 1 teaspoon low-calorie dressing	446	12.5
Bedtime drink A cup of chocolate: 1 tablespoon Hershey's chocolate syrup with milk from allowance	53	0.0
Total	**1,487**	**35.7**

*COTTAGE CHEESE AND RAISIN SANDWICH
Serves 1

¼   cup cottage cheese with pineapple
2   tablespoons raisins
2   slices of whole-wheat bread

Mix the cottage cheese with raisins and spread on bread.

*MACARONI AND VEGETABLE CHEESE BAKE
Serves 1

¼   cup whole-wheat macaroni
⅔   cup frozen mixed vegetables
1   tablespoon whole-wheat flour
½   cup skim milk (from allowance)
1   teaspoon diet margarine
     Salt and pepper to taste
¼   teaspoon prepared mustard
¼   cup grated Cheddar cheese

Boil the macaroni in lightly salted water for 12 minutes, or until just tender. Drain well. Cook the vegetables as directed and drain. Put the flour, milk, and margarine in a saucepan and heat, stirring constantly, until it boils and thickens. Season with salt and pepper. Add the mustard and half the cheese. Stir the macaroni and vegetables into the sauce. Put in an ovenproof dish. Top with remaining cheese. Cook in a moderately hot oven (400°F) for 20 minutes, or until the cheese is browned.

1,500-Calorie Menu #6 no Fiber-Filler

	Calories	Fiber (g)
Daily allowance: 2 cups skim milk, an orange, and an apple or pear	366	8.2
Breakfast ¾ cup Kellogg's 40% Branflakes with milk from allowance	79	4.4
Midmorning snack 1 Nature Valley Honey 'N Oats Granola Bar	150	1.0
Lunch 1 cup Heinz chili con carne with beans	340	23.0
After-school snack 2 graham crackers	54	1.4
Evening meal *Oven-Baked Chicken and Chips 2 medium tomatoes Orange from allowance	476	6.8
Bedtime snack and drink 1 graham cracker 2 tablespoons orange soda mixed with ½ cup milk from allowance	27	0.7
Total	**1,492**	**45.5**

*OVEN-BAKED CHICKEN AND CHIPS   *Serves 1*

1   chicken leg and thigh
     Salt and pepper to taste
½   cup frozen french fries

Season the chicken well with salt and pepper and wrap in foil.
Bake in a hot oven (425°F) for 45 minutes or until tender.
Place the french fries on a baking tray and bake with the
chicken for the last 15 to 20 minutes. Unwrap the chicken and
remove and discard the skin. Serve with the french fries.

1,500-Calorie Menu #7 no Fiber-Filler

	Calories	Fiber (g)
Daily allowance: 2 cups skim milk, an orange, and an apple or pear	366	8.2
Breakfast 1 cup Kellogg's Raisin Bran with milk from allowance Orange from allowance	130	10.3
Midmorning snack 3 tablespoons raisins	173	3.4
Lunch *1 Peanut Butter and Strawberry Bagel (2 halves) 1 medium carrot, cut into sticks Apple or pear from allowance	399	7.5
After-school snack 2 graham crackers	54	1.4

Evening meal

4 ounces cod or haddock fillets brushed with 1 teaspoon diet margarine and broiled		
1 tomato, halved, grilled without fat		
½ mashed potato (no butter)		
½ cup frozen peas, cooked	332	10.2

Bedtime drink

A cup of chocolate: 1 tablespoon Hershey's chocolate syrup with skim milk from allowance	53	0.0
Total	**1,507**	**41.0**

*PEANUT BUTTER AND STRAWBERRY
BAGEL   *Serves 1*

1   whole-wheat bagel
2   tablespoons peanut butter
1   tablespoon diet strawberry jam
¼   cup sliced fresh strawberries

Split bagel. Spread one half of bagel with peanut butter. Spread the other half with jam and top with sliced strawberries. Put halves together.

1,500-Calorie Menu #8 no Fiber-Filler

	Calories	Fiber (g)
Daily allowance: 2 cups skim milk, an orange, and an apple or pear	366	8.2

Breakfast
¾ cup Kellogg's All-Bran with 1
    tablespoon raisins and milk from
    allowance
1 RyKrisp cracker spread with 1
    teaspoon diet margarine   166   14.2

Midmorning snack
1 Nature Valley Honey 'N Oats Granola
    Bar
Orange from allowance   150   1.0

Lunch
1 egg, poached and served on 1 slice of
    whole-wheat bread, toasted and
    spread with 1 teaspoon diet margarine
*Apricot Yogurt Dessert   408   10.3

After-school snack
1 cup fresh strawberries
25 grapes   131   4.3

Evening meal
*Liver-and-Mushroom-Filled Potato
½ cup canned tomatoes
¾ cup cabbage, boiled   290   9.2

Bedtime snack
Apple or pear from allowance

                                   Total   1,511   47.2

*APRICOT YOGURT DESSERT   *Serves 1*

1   cup plain low-fat yogurt
8   halves dried apricots (no-need-to-soak variety), chopped
1   teaspoon honey
1   tablespoon bran

Mix the yogurt, apricots, and honey. Let stand for at least 30 minutes to allow flavors to blend. Serve sprinkled with bran.

*LIVER-AND-MUSHROOM-FILLED POTATO   *Serves 1*

1   large potato
2   ounces chopped chicken liver
1   tablespoon finely chopped onion
¼   cup sliced mushrooms
¼   cup peas, cooked
⅓   cup skim milk from allowance
    Salt and pepper to taste
    Dash of Worcestershire sauce

Scrub the potato well and bake (see page 20). Meanwhile, put the chicken liver, onion, mushrooms, peas, and milk in a small pan. Heat to a simmer, cover, and cook gently for 5 minutes. Cut the potato in half lengthwise and scoop out some of the flesh. Mix the flesh with the chicken liver mixture. Season with salt and pepper and add the Worcestershire sauce. Pile back into the potato jackets. Heat in the oven for 5 to 10 minutes, if necessary.

1,500-Calorie Menu #9 no Fiber-Filler

	Calories	Fiber (g)
Daily allowance: 2 cups skim milk, an orange, and an apple or pear	366	8.2
Breakfast 2 cups Kellogg's All-Bran topped with ½ sliced banana with milk from allowance	170	18.2
Midmorning snack 1 small (¾-ounce) package of potato chips	114	1.0
Lunch *Tuna and Celery Sandwich 1 medium tomato, sliced Apple or pear from allowance 2 graham crackers	322	6.0
After-school snack 1 Fibermed Apple/Currant Biscuit with 1 tablespoon low-calorie fruit preserves Orange from allowance	87	5.0
Evening meal *Chicken Risotto 2 RyKrisp crackers with 2 tablespoons cream cheese	353	7.4
Bedtime drink Milk shake: 1 tablespoon Hershey's chocolate syrup with milk from allowance	53	0.0
Total	**1,465**	**45.8**

*TUNA AND CELERY SANDWICH   *Serves 1*

2   tablespoons water-packed tuna, drained and flaked
1   celery stalk, finely chopped
1   tablespoon diet mayonnaise
2   slices of whole-wheat bread

Mash the tuna with a fork, then mix with the celery and mayonnaise. Spread the tuna mixture on one slice of bread and top with the second slice.

*CHICKEN RISOTTO   *Serves 1*

¼   cup brown rice
1   small onion, finely chopped
5   mushrooms, sliced
1   small green pepper, seeded and chopped
1   tomato, chopped
½   chicken bouillon cube
    Pinch of rosemary
    Salt and pepper to taste
¼   cup cooked diced chicken

Put the rice, onion, mushrooms, green pepper, and tomato in a pan. Dissolve the ½ bouillon cube in 1 cup boiling water and pour into the pan. Bring to a boil and add the rosemary and salt and pepper. Stir well, reduce heat, cover, and simmer until the stock is absorbed and the rice is tender, about 25 minutes. Stir the chicken into the rice mixture and heat through gently. Serve hot.

1,500-Calorie Menu #10 no Fiber-Filler

	Calories	Fiber (g)
Daily allowance: 2 cups skim milk, an orange, and an apple or pear	366	8.2
Breakfast 1 cup Kellogg's Raisin Bran with milk from allowance Orange from allowance	130	10.3
Midmorning snack 1 Fibermed Apple/Currant Biscuit	60	5.0
Lunch 2 frozen fish sticks, baked ⅔ cup canned baked beans in tomato sauce mixed with 1 tablespoon bran Apple or pear from allowance	287	17.7
After-school snack 2 tablespoons Planter's Soy Nuts	126	1.3
Evening meal *Cheese and Potato Pie *Raisin-Stuffed Baked Apple	445	11.0
Bedtime drink A cup of chocolate: 1 tablespoon Hershey's chocolate syrup with milk from allowance	53	0.0
Total	**1,467**	**53.5**

*CHEESE AND POTATO PIE   *Serves 1*

1   large potato, scrubbed and sliced
1   small onion, peeled and thinly sliced
¼   cup grated Cheddar cheese
¼   cup canned corn
    Salt and pepper to taste
½   cup skim milk from allowance

Arrange half the potato slices in the bottom of a small oven-proof dish. Top with the onion and half the cheese. Add the corn. Season with salt and pepper. Repeat the layers, using up the remaining potato, onion, and cheese. Heat the milk. Pour over the cheese and vegetables. Cover and bake at 325°F for 1 hour. Serve hot.

*RAISIN-STUFFED BAKED APPLE   *Serves 1*

1   cooking apple
2   tablespoons raisins
¼   cup diet raspberry soda

Wash the apple and remove the core, leaving a hole for the filling. Cut through the skin around the center of the apple with a sharp knife to keep it from bursting during cooking. Put the apple in a small ovenproof dish. Fill with raisins. Pour soda around apple. Bake at 325°F with the Cheese and Potato Pie for 45 minutes, or until the apple is tender right through but not overcooked. Serve hot or cold.

F-Plan Menus for Freezer-Owner Cooks

The inventor of the home freezer inadvertently invented the best dieting aid ever. Here's how to use it to maximum advantage, whether you cook and store F-Plan meals (pages 224–265) or prefer to buy and store frozen convenience foods and follow the menus in the chapter on "Canned and Packaged F-Plan" (page 139).

An enormously helpful way of ensuring that you stick to your diet is to plan ahead and prepare and store most of the foods you will need. One of the many advantages of this strategy is that when you start dieting you will be able to spend much less time in the kitchen, where the cookie jar, bread box, and refrigerator all seem to beckon to you, weakening your resolve. You are off to a head start if you stock your freezer with most if not all the sauces, soups, pizzas, flans, and meat dishes, packed in individual portions; you will then avoid all temptation to eat the wrong thing because you did not have time to shop for and cook the right thing.

The recipes for all the freezer dishes are given before the menus and not scattered throughout as in other sections, because freezer owners usually "batch" cook in advance and then store the food until the day on which it is to be eaten. Recipes for four savory sauces have been included, which can be used to liven up fish, meat, and eggs with minimal effort. In addition to the home-cooked frozen foods in the menus, one or two other foods commonly found in freezers—for example, ice cream and frozen fruit, vegetables, and fish—have been included. Should you be concerned that all the foods in these menus come from the freezer and nothing is fresh, it will be reassuring to know that the menus follow all the basic F-Plan diet rules (page 12) and contain the daily allowances of one portion of Fiber-Filler, an orange and an apple or pear, and 1 cup skim milk. The menus also contain fresh bread, other fresh fruits, fresh vegetables, eggs, cheese, and some fresh meat.

The menus are divided up into two parts: approximately 1,000 calories and 1,250 calories daily, all providing 35 to 60 g fiber.

Instructions have been included for reheating the frozen dishes in a microwave oven, as this is a particularly quick and convenient way of cooking or reheating frozen food.

Special Diet Notes

1. Begin by deciding which daily calorie total will give you a satisfactory weight loss (page 15).

2. Select the menus from your chosen daily calorie total for at least one week, preferably two or more, so that you can plan which dishes you need to prepare in advance and freeze. Remember to vary the menus and hence the foods to ensure that you are eating all the nutrients you need for good health.

3. Do as much cooking as you can before starting the diet and have the dishes frozen in single portions.

4. Begin each day with Fiber-Filler (recipe on page 13) from the daily allowance, which you can prepare in batch quantities too, if you wish.

5. Drink as much tea and coffee without sugar (artificial sweeteners can be used) as you wish each day, but remember to use only the skim milk from the daily allowance. In addition, drink as much water and drinks labeled "low-calorie" as you wish. Alcoholic drinks have not been included in these menus. Should you find it impossible to follow a diet that does not allow an occasional alcoholic drink, and if you are achieving a good weight loss, then you could try allowing yourself an increased calorie intake by selecting drinks from the chart (page 266). However, it would be advisable to limit these to a daily total of 200 calories, and if your weight loss stops then it will be necessary to leave out the drinks.

SAUCES

TOMATO SAUCE   *6 portions*

(34 calories, 2.5 g fiber per portion)

4   cups canned tomatoes
1   large onion, peeled and chopped
1   large carrot, peeled and grated
1   celery stalk, cut up
1   bay leaf
     Salt and pepper to taste
¼   cup bran

Put all the ingredients in a medium-size saucepan with 1 cup water, bring to a boil, reduce the heat, and simmer for 20 minutes. Remove the bay leaf and purée the sauce, either through a sieve or in a blender. Season to taste.

To freeze
Let cool; divide equally among six or more plastic bags or individual freezer containers, seal, label, and freeze.

To serve
Leave at room temperature for at least 3 hours, turn into a saucepan, and heat gently until piping hot.

or
Turn out frozen onto a dish, cover with plastic wrap, and microwave on full power for 1¼ minutes; remove from the oven and break up by using a fork. Microwave on full power for a further 1¼ minutes.

BARBECUE SAUCE   *6 portions*

(40 calories, 2 g fiber per portion)

1   cup unsweetened apple sauce
⅓   cup tomato purée
2   teaspoons vinegar
2   teaspoons Worcestershire sauce
4   teaspoons sugar
10   small mushrooms, finely chopped
¼   cup bran
     Salt and pepper to taste

Put all ingredients in a medium-size saucepan with 2 cups water, bring to a boil, reduce the heat, and simmer for 20 minutes. Season to taste.

To freeze
Let cool; divide equally among six or eight plastic bags or individual freezer containers, seal, label, and freeze.

To serve
Leave at room temperature for at least 2½ hours, turn out into a saucepan, and heat gently until piping hot.

or
Turn out frozen portion onto a dish, cover with plastic wrap, and microwave on full power for 1¼ minutes; remove from the oven and break up using a fork. Microwave on full power for a further 1¼ minutes.

SWEET AND SOUR SAUCE   *4 portions*

(83 calories, 2.4 g fiber per portion)

1   cup juice-packed pineapple chunks
1   tablespoon honey
1   tablespoon vinegar
2   tablespoons cornstarch
3   tablespoons soy sauce
1   green pepper, cut into thin strips
1   medium carrot, peeled and cut into thin strips
¼   cup bran
     Salt and pepper to taste

   Drain the pineapple, reserving the juice. Add water to the juice to make 1 cup and put in a saucepan with the honey and vinegar. Mix the cornstarch and soy sauce together, add to the water, and bring to a boil, stirring constantly. When it thickens, add the vegetables, bran, and pineapple, reduce the heat, and simmer for 20 to 25 minutes.

To freeze
Let cool; divide equally among four or more plastic bags or individual freezer containers, seal, label, and freeze.

To serve
Leave at room temperature for at least 3 hours, turn out into a saucepan, and heat gently until piping hot.

or
Turn out frozen portion onto a dish, cover with plastic wrap, and microwave on full power for 1½ minutes; remove from the oven and break up using a fork. Microwave on full power for a further 1½ minutes.

CURRY SAUCE   *6 portions*

(106 calories, 4.1 g fiber per portion)

1   large onion, peeled and chopped
1   large celery stalk, finely chopped
1   teaspoon oil
1   tablespoon curry powder
2   tablespoons pickle relish
1   apple, cored and chopped
½   cup dried lentils
2   tablespoons raisins
1   tablespoon lemon juice

Gently fry the onion and celery in the oil for 3 to 4 minutes. Add the curry powder and pickle relish and mix well. Add 2 cups water and bring to a boil. Add the apple, lentils, raisins, and lemon juice, bring back to a boil, reduce the heat, and simmer for 25 to 30 minutes, or until the lentils are soft.

To freeze
Let cool; divide among six or more small containers (for example, empty yogurt cartons). Cover and seal, label, and freeze.

To serve
Thaw at room temperature for at least 3 hours, empty into a saucepan, and heat gently until piping hot.

or
Turn out frozen portion onto a dish, cover with plastic wrap, and microwave on full power for 1½ minutes. Remove and break up using a fork. Microwave on full power for a further 1¼ minutes.

SOUPS

CREAMY PEA SOUP   *5 portions*

(85 calories, 7 g fiber per portion)

1   pound fresh or frozen peas (3½ cups)
1   large onion, peeled and chopped
1   tablespoon chopped fresh mint or 1 teaspoon dried mint
¼   cup bran
3½   cups chicken bouillon (made from 2 chicken bouillon
     cubes)
1   teaspoon sugar
     Salt and pepper to taste
2   tablespoons nonfat dry milk powder

Put the peas, onion, mint, bran, bouillon, and sugar in a sauce-pan. Season with salt and pepper. Bring to a boil, cover, and simmer for 30 minutes. Purée in a blender or push through a sieve. Blend the milk powder with a little of the soup and return to the saucepan with the remaining soup. Reheat gently without boiling. Sprinkle with bran.

To freeze
Let cool; divide equally among five 1-cup containers. Cover, label, and freeze.

To serve
Thaw at room temperature for 2 hours, turn into a saucepan, and heat gently until piping hot.

or
Turn out frozen portion into a bowl, cover with plastic wrap, and microwave on full power for 2 minutes; remove and break up using a fork. Microwave on full power for a further 2 minutes, until piping hot.

CARROT AND LENTIL SOUP   *4 portions*

(133 calories, 7.6 g fiber per portion)

2½ cups chicken bouillon, made with 1 bouillon cube
3½ carrots, scrubbed and sliced
½   cup lentils
1   large onion, peeled and chopped
1   celery stalk, chopped
2   teaspoons lemon juice
1   tablespoon chopped parsley
     Salt and pepper to taste

In a large saucepan bring the chicken bouillon to a boil. Add the carrots, lentils, onion, and celery and simmer for 25 minutes, or until the vegetables are tender. Remove from the heat and purée through a sieve or in a blender. Return to the saucepan and add the lemon juice and parsley. Season with salt and pepper.

To freeze
Let cool; divide equally among four 1-cup containers, cover, label, and freeze.

To serve
Thaw at room temperature for at least 1½ hours. Empty soup into a saucepan and heat gently until piping hot.

or
Turn out freezer portion into a bowl and cover with plastic wrap and microwave on full power for 5 minutes, stirring after 2 and 4 minutes.

CORN POTAGE   *7 portions*

(148 calories, 5.9 g fiber per portion)

3   cups chicken bouillon, made with 2 chicken bouillon
     cubes
5   large potatoes, scrubbed and diced
1   large onion, peeled and chopped
1½ cups canned corn
10 mushrooms, sliced
1   green pepper, seeded and chopped
2   tablespoons nonfat dry milk powder
     Salt and pepper to taste
2   tablespoons bran

Put the bouillon in a large saucepan and bring to a boil. Add
the potatoes, onion, corn, mushrooms, and green pepper and
simmer for 30 minutes, or until the vegetables are soft. Remove from the heat and let cool slightly; gradually stir in the
milk powder. Season. Return to the heat and gently bring back
to a boil. Sprinkle with bran.

To freeze
Let cool. Divide equally among seven 1-cup containers, cover
and label, and freeze.

To serve
Thaw at room temperature for at least 2½ hours, empty into a
saucepan, and heat gently until piping hot.

or
Turn out frozen portion into a bowl, cover with plastic wrap,
and microwave on full power for 5 minutes, stirring after 2 and
4 minutes.

MAIN DISHES

ZUCCHINI AND CORN FLAN   *6 portions*

(228 calories and 4.8 g fiber per portion)

PASTRY
1½ cups whole-wheat flour
6   tablespoons diet margarine

FILLING
1   large onion, peeled and thinly sliced
½   cup canned corn
½   pound zucchini, thinly sliced
1   egg
½   cup skim milk
¼   teaspoon dry mustard
     Salt and pepper to taste
¼   cup grated Cheddar cheese

Put the flour in a bowl and cut in the margarine until the mixture resembles bread crumbs. Stir in 3 tablespoons water and gather dough together into a ball. Roll out the pastry (between two sheets of waxed paper for easier handling) and line an 8-inch pie tin. Line the flan pastry with waxed paper and weight with ½ cup dry beans. Bake at 425°F for 10 minutes. Lift out the paper and beans and return the pastry to the oven for 5 minutes. Turn the oven down to 350°F. Arrange the onion and corn in the bottom of the pastry. Arrange the zucchini slices in overlapping circles on top of the corn and onion. Beat the egg, milk, mustard, and salt and pepper together. Pour into the pastry. Bake in the oven for 15 minutes, then remove. Sprinkle the grated cheese over the top and return to the oven for 20 minutes, or until the egg mixture is set and the cheese browned.

To freeze
Let cool quickly, then cut into six equal pieces. Wrap each piece in foil, label, and freeze.

To serve
Loosen foil wrapping and thaw at room temperature for 3 hours.

MEAT AND VEGETABLE LOAF   *6 portions*

(215 calories, 5.3 g fiber per portion)

½   cup lentils
¾   pound ground beef
1   large onion, peeled and chopped
1¼ cups grated carrots
¾   cup whole-wheat bread crumbs
3   tablespoons tomato purée
½   teaspoon dry basil
¼   teaspoon garlic powder
    Salt and pepper to taste

Bring the lentils to a boil in 2 cups water, then simmer gently for 25 minutes, or until the lentils are soft; drain and reserve. Preheat the oven to 350°F. Lightly grease a 1-quart loaf pan. Thoroughly mix lentils and remaining ingredients in a large bowl. Put the mixture in the loaf pan; press down firmly, using the back of a spoon. Bake in the middle of the oven for 1½ hours, or until the loaf is brown and firm to the touch.

To freeze
Let cool in the tin; turn out and cut into six slices. Pack slices in six plastic bags or individual freezer containers; seal, label, and freeze.

To serve
Thaw at room temperature for at least 3½ hours; then either heat through in a hot oven or heat under the grill.

or
Turn out the frozen slices onto a dish, cover with plastic wrap, and microwave on full power for 2 minutes; turn over and microwave for a further 2 minutes.

SARDINE AND TOMATO PIZZA *6 portions*

(244 calories, 5.3 g fiber per portion)

2   cups whole-wheat flour
1   teaspoon salt
1   tablespoon diet margarine
1   envelope dry yeast

TOPPING
1   tablespoon tomato purée
1   (3¾-ounce) can of Underwood sardines in tomato sauce
1   large onion, peeled and thinly sliced
3   tomatoes, sliced
¾   cup grated mozzarella cheese
½   teaspoon dried basil
2   tablespoons bran

Put the flour, salt, and margarine in a large mixing bowl and rub together until the mixture resembles bread crumbs. Stir in the yeast and add ½ cup warm water to form a soft dough. Knead the dough for 5 to 7 minutes, until smooth. Leave to rise in a bowl for 30 minutes, or until it has doubled in size. Divide the dough into 5 portions; roll out each one to fit a 6-inch round freezer container. Spread the tomato purée over them. Mash the sardines together with their sauce and place evenly over the tomato purée. Place the onion, tomato, and cheese on each pizza, and sprinkle a little basil and 1 teaspoon bran over each pizza.

To freeze
Freeze, uncovered, and when frozen, place with the container in a plastic bag, seal and label, and freeze.

To serve
Defrost at room temperature for at least 2 hours and bake in a preheated 400°F oven 15 minutes, or until base is crusty.

BEEF AND BEAN CASSEROLE   *6 portions*

(198 calories, 5.3 g fiber per portion)

¾   pound stew beef (lean chuck), cut into 1-inch cubes
1   large onion, peeled and chopped
1   large carrot, peeled and sliced
1   cup canned baked beans in tomato sauce
2   tablespoons pearl barley
1   cup beef bouillon (made from 1 bouillon cube)
1   teaspoon Worcestershire sauce
1   teaspoon vinegar
    Salt and pepper to taste

Preheat the oven to 325°F. Put the meat in a 1-quart ovenproof dish with the onion, carrot, baked beans, and barley. Mix together the beef bouillon, Worcestershire sauce, and vinegar and pour over the meat. Season with salt and pepper. Cover and bake in the middle of the oven for 2 hours, or until the meat and carrot are tender.

To freeze
Let cool; then divide equally among six plastic bags or individual freezer containers. Seal, label, and freeze.

To serve

Thaw at room temperature for at least 2 hours, empty into a saucepan, and heat gently until piping hot.

or

Turn out frozen portion onto a dish. Cover with plastic wrap and microwave on full power for 2 minutes; remove from the microwave and break up, using a fork. Microwave on full power for 1½ minutes.

CHILI CON CARNE   *4 portions*

(205 calories, 8.4 g fiber per portion)

½   cup kidney beans, soaked in water overnight
1   large onion, peeled and chopped
½   pound ground beef
2   large celery stalks, finely chopped
10   mushrooms, sliced
2   tablespoons tomato purée
1   to 2 teaspoons chili powder, or to taste
2   cups canned tomatoes
     Salt and pepper to taste

Bring the kidney beans to a boil in lightly salted water and boil rapidly for 15 minutes; remove from the heat and drain. Gently fry the onion and ground beef, without added fat, for 2 to 3 minutes. To the meat mixture add the celery, mushrooms, tomato purée, and chili powder, and mix thoroughly until the ingredients are evenly distributed. Pour in the tomatoes and ½ cup water and add the kidney beans. Stir until the mixture is boiling. Reduce heat, cover, and leave to simmer gently for approximately 1 hour, or until the kidney beans are tender. Season to taste.

To freeze
Let cool; then divide equally among four plastic bags or four individual freezer containers. Seal, label, and freeze.

To serve
Thaw at room temperature for at least 2 hours. Empty into a saucepan and heat gently until piping hot.

or
Turn out frozen portion onto a dish. Cover with plastic wrap and microwave on full power for 1¼ minutes; remove from the microwave and break up, using a fork. Microwave on full power for a further 1½ minutes.

PORK WITH PRUNES   *5 portions*

(283 calories, 7.8 g fiber per portion)

1   pound boneless lean pork roast (Invisible Chef), fat removed, cut into 1-inch cubes
10   dried prunes, soaked overnight and drained
¼   cup raisins
1   apple, cored and chopped
2   tablespoons sweet pickle relish

Preheat the oven to 350°F. Put the meat in a 1-quart ovenproof dish with the prunes, raisins, and apple. Mix the relish with 1 cup water and pour over the meat. Cover and bake in the middle of the oven for 1 hour, or until the meat is tender.

To freeze
Let cool; then divide equally among five plastic bags or five individual freezer containers. Seal, label, and freeze.

To serve
Thaw at room temperature for at least 2 hours, empty into a saucepan, and heat gently until piping hot.

or

Turn out frozen portion onto a dish, cover with plastic wrap, and microwave on full power for 1½ minutes. Remove from the microwave and break up, using a fork. Microwave on full power for a further 1½ minutes.

PAPRIKA CHICKEN   *4 portions*

(270 calories, 7.5 g fiber per portion)

¼   cup dry lima beans, soaked overnight and drained
1½ pounds chicken, cut up, skin removed
¾   cup frozen corn
3   tablespoons brown rice
1   (1-pound) can of tomatoes
½   cup chicken bouillon (made from ½ bouillon cube)
1   tablespoon vinegar
¼   teaspoon paprika

Preheat the oven to 375°F. Put the lima beans and chicken pieces in a 1½-quart ovenproof dish with the corn, rice, and tomatoes. Mix together the bouillon, vinegar, and paprika and pour over the chicken. Cover and bake in the middle of the oven for 50 to 55 minutes, or until the chicken and rice are tender.
To freeze
Let cool; then divide equally among four plastic bags or four individual freezer containers. Seal, label, and freeze.
To serve
Thaw at room temperature for at least 2 hours, empty into an ovenproof dish, and reheat at 400°F for 35 to 40 minutes.
or
Turn out rozen portion onto a dish, cover with plastic wrap, and microwave on full power for 2 minutes. Take the chicken out and turn it over. Cook for 2 minutes on full power. Repeat this two more times.

LAMB WITH SPLIT PEAS   *4 portions*

(263 calories, 5.5 g fiber per portion)

½   pound lean shoulder of lamb, cut into 1-inch cubes
½   cup dried split peas, soaked in water overnight
1   large onion, peeled and chopped
2½ large carrots, peeled and sliced
2   bay leaves
½   teaspoon ground nutmeg
1½ cups beef bouillon (made from 1 bouillon cube)

Preheat the oven to 325°F. Gently fry the lamb in a nonstick pan, without added fat, until lightly browned. Drain off and discard any fat that has cooked out of the meat. Put meat in a 1-quart ovenproof dish with the remaining ingredients. Cover the dish and bake in the middle of the oven for 2 to 2¼ hours, until the meat and carrots are tender.

To freeze
Let cool; then divide equally among four plastic bags or four individual freezer containers. Seal, label, and freeze.

To serve
Thaw at room temperature for at least 2 hours, empty into a saucepan, and heat gently until piping hot.

or
Turn out frozen portion onto a dish, cover with plastic wrap, and microwave on full power for 1¼ minutes. Remove and break up, using a fork. Microwave on full power for a further 1¼ minutes.

DESSERTS

PEAR AND APRICOT MOUSSE   *8 portions*

(98 calories, 2 g fiber per portion)

1   (16-ounce) can of juice-packed pears
1   (16-ounce) can of juice-packed apricots
3   eggs, separated
1   teaspoon honey
1   envelope or 3 teaspoons powdered gelatin
2   tablespoons bran

Reserve 3 tablespoons juice from the can of pears and purée the pears and apricots with the remaining juice. Beat the egg yolks and honey with 1 teaspoon hot water until pale and creamy. Put the gelatin in a small heatproof bowl with the reserved juice. Stand the bowl in a saucepan of water and heat until the gelatin is dissolved. Let cool slightly; stir into the egg yolk mixture with the fruit purée. Beat the egg whites until stiff and gently fold into the mixture. Sprinkle bran on mousse before serving.

To freeze
Divide the mousse equally among eight 1-cup containers (for example, cottage cheese cartons). Cover, label, and freeze.

To serve
Thaw in the refrigerator for 2½ to 3 hours.

PLUM CHARLOTTE   *6 portions*

(113 calories, 3.3 g fiber per portion)

1   pound plums, pitted
½   cup whole-wheat bread crumbs
¼   cup granola
¼   cup bran
¼   teaspoon ground cinnamon
     Grated rind of 1 orange
6   tablespoons fresh orange juice
2   tablespoons brown sugar

Divide half the plums equally among six individual soufflé dishes or custard cups. Mix the bread crumbs, granola, bran, cinnamon, and orange rind. Sprinkle half this mixture over the plums. Cover with the remaining plums and top with the remaining bread crumb mixture. Mix the orange juice with the sugar and spoon an equal amount over the top of each charlotte. Stand the dishes on a baking tray and bake at 350°F for 30 minutes, until the top is crisp and browned. Serve hot.

To freeze
Cool as quickly as possible, cover with foil, label, and freeze.

To serve
Thaw at room temperature for 2 to 3 hours, then heat through in the oven at 400°F for about 15 minutes, or until hot.

RHUBARB AND BREAD PUDDING   *6 portions*

(131 calories, 3.1 g fiber per portion)

4   cups rhubarb, cut into 1-inch pieces
4   slices of whole-wheat bread, cubed
2   tablespoons raisins
3   tablespoons brown sugar
½   teaspoon ground ginger
1½ cups skim milk
2   eggs

Preheat the oven to 350°F. Divide half the rhubarb among six individual baking dishes and cover with half the bread. Sprinkle the raisins over the bread and repeat the rhubarb and bread layers once more. Beat together the sugar, ginger, milk, and eggs, and pour over the rhubarb and bread. Let stand for 20 to 30 minutes. Bake in the oven for 30 minutes, until the custard is set and rhubarb is soft.

To freeze
Let cool, cover, label, and freeze.

To serve
Thaw at room temperature for 2 hours, uncover, and reheat at 400°F for about 15 to 20 minutes, or until heated through.

TUTTI-FRUTTI ICE CREAM　*6 portions*

(112 calories, 5.7 g fiber per portion)

2	tablespoons slivered almonds
2	tablespoons whole-wheat bread crumbs
1	cup plain low-fat yogurt
9	dried apricot halves, finely chopped
2	tablespoons raisins
3	egg whites
6	tablespoons brown sugar

Toast the almonds and bread crumbs until golden brown. Add to the yogurt with the apricots and raisins. Beat the egg whites until stiff, add the sugar, and beat again until stiff. Fold the yogurt mixture into the egg whites and pour into a rigid plastic container (for example, an ice cream carton). Freeze until just solid. Cut into six equal portions, wrap individually in plastic wrap, and put in a plastic bag; put in the freezer.

To serve
Transfer to refrigerator for 20 to 30 minutes before serving, to allow the ice cream to soften slightly.

BLUEBERRY AND APPLE CRUMBLE   *5 portions*

(187 calories, 6.3 g fiber per portion)

CRUMBLE TOPPING
1   cup whole-wheat flour
¼   cup diet margarine
2   tablespoons soft brown sugar
¼   cup dry coconut

FILLING
1   cup blueberries
2   apples, cored and sliced
1   teaspoon honey

Put the flour and margarine in a mixing bowl and cut together until the mixture resembles bread crumbs. Stir in the sugar and coconut. Mix the blueberries, apple slices, and honey and divide among five individual custard cups. Sprinkle on the crumble topping.

To freeze
Cover the uncooked crumbles, label, and freeze.

To serve
Defrost at room temperature for 2 hours; uncover and cook in a preheated oven (400°F) for about 20 minutes, or until crumble topping is browned.

1,000-Calorie Menu #1

	Calories	Fiber (g)
Daily allowance: Fiber-Filler, 1 cup skim milk, an orange, and an apple or pear	450	23.0
Breakfast Half portion of Fiber-Filler with milk from allowance Orange from allowance		
Lunch 1 portion Corn Potage (page 232) ¼ cup water-packed tuna, flaked (Mix the tuna into the soup, then heat in a saucepan. Serve hot.) Apple or pear from allowance	211	5.9
Evening meal 1 portion Pork with Prunes (page 238) 9 frozen Brussels sprouts, cooked 1 medium carrot, cooked and sliced 1 portion Pear and Apricot Mousse (page 241)	426	12.2
Snack Remaining Fiber-Filler with milk from allowance		
Total	**1,087**	**41.1**

1,000-Calorie Menu #2

	Calories	Fiber (g)
Daily allowance: Fiber-Filler, 1 cup skim milk, an orange, and an apple or pear	450	23.0
Breakfast Half portion of Fiber-Filler with milk from allowance Apple or pear from allowance		
Lunch 1 egg, poached and served on 1 slice of whole-wheat bread, toasted and spread with 1 teaspoon diet margarine 1 portion Tutti-Frutti Ice Cream (page 244)	271	6.9
Evening meal 1 portion Chili con Carne (page 237) ¾ cup cabbage, cooked 1 large carrot Orange from allowance	262	14.7
Snack Remaining Fiber-Filler with milk from allowance		
Total	**983**	**44.6**

1,000-Calorie Menu #3

	Calories	Fiber (g)
Daily allowance: Fiber-Filler, 1 cup skim milk, an orange, and an apple or pear	450	23.0
Breakfast Half portion of Fiber-Filler with milk from allowance Orange from allowance		
Lunch 1 portion Carrot and Lentil Soup (page 231) 4 whole-wheat crackers 1 ounce mozzarella cheese Apple or pear from allowance	276	9.3
Evening meal 2 ounces ham steak, broiled, without fat added 1 portion Sweet and Sour Sauce (page 228) ½ cup canned corn ½ cup fresh strawberries	312	7.6
Snack Remaining Fiber-Filler with milk from allowance		
Total	**1,009**	**37.9**

1,000-Calorie Menu #4

	Calories	Fiber (g)
Daily allowance: Fiber-Filler, 1 cup skim milk, an orange, and an apple or pear	450	23.0
Breakfast Half portion of Fiber-Filler with milk from allowance Apple or pear from allowance		
Lunch 2 ounces hamburger, broiled, served on 2 slices of whole-wheat bread with 1 tablespoon pickle relish and 1 medium tomato, sliced Orange from allowance	266	4.2
Evening meal ½ package Gorton's Sole with Lemon Butter ¾ cup frozen mixed vegetables 1 cup fresh blueberries sweetened with 1 teaspoon sugar	341	13.0
Snack Remaining Fiber-Filler with milk from allowance		
Total	**1,057**	**40.2**

1,000-Calorie Menu #5

	Calories	Fiber (g)
Daily allowance: Fiber-Filler, 1 cup skim milk, an orange, and an apple or pear	450	23.0
Breakfast Half portion of Fiber-Filler with milk from allowance Orange from allowance		
Lunch 1 portion Creamy Pea Soup (page 230) 1 slice bacon, broiled and crumbled over the soup 2 whole-wheat crackers Apple or pear from allowance	182	7.8
Evening meal 1 portion Lamb with Split Peas (page 240) 12 Brussels sprouts, cooked ½ cup potatoes, boiled and mashed with a little skim milk from allowance, no butter 12 green grapes	436	11.2
Snack Remaining Fiber-Filler with milk from allowance		
Total	**1,068**	**42.0**

1,000-Calorie Menu #6

	Calories	Fiber (g)
Daily allowance: Fiber-Filler, 1 cup skim milk, an orange, and an apple or pear	450	23.0
Breakfast Half portion of Fiber-Filler with milk from allowance 12 green grapes	37	0.5
Lunch 1 portion Meat and Vegetable Loaf (page 234) heated with 1 portion Tomato Sauce (page 226) ½ cup shredded white cabbage, mixed with ⅔ cup grated carrot and 1 tablespoon diet mayonnaise Orange from allowance	334	10.6
Evening meal 1 portion Corn Potage (page 232) 2 ounces frozen shrimps, thawed (Heat the soup with the shrimps until piping hot.) 1 Fibermed Apple/Currant Biscuit Apple or pear from allowance	238	10.9
Snack Remaining Fiber-Filler with milk from allowance		
Total	**1,059**	**45.0**

1,000-Calorie Menu #7

	Calories	Fiber (g)
Daily allowance: Fiber-Filler, 1 cup skim milk, an orange, and an apple or pear	450	23.0
Breakfast Half portion of Fiber-Filler with milk from allowance		
Lunch 1 portion Zucchini and Corn Flan (page 233) 1 medium carrot, cut into sticks 1 celery stalk, cut into sticks Orange from allowance	252	6.7
Evening meal 1 portion Paprika Chicken (page 239) 1 cup chopped frozen spinach, cooked without butter 2 whole-wheat crackers with 2 tablespoons cottage cheese with pineapple, topped with 2 tablespoons chopped green pepper Apple or pear from allowance	372	18.5
Snack Remaining Fiber-Filler with milk from allowance		
Total	**1,074**	**48.2**

1,000-Calorie Menu #8

	Calories	Fiber (g)
Daily allowance: Fiber-Filler, 1 cup skim milk, an orange, and an apple or pear	450	23.0
Breakfast Half portion of Fiber-Filler with milk from allowance		
Lunch Curried egg on toast: 1 large slice of whole-wheat bread, toasted and topped with 1 poached egg and 1 portion Curry Sauce (page 229), heated Apple or pear from allowance	249	5.3
Evening meal 1 portion Meat and Vegetable Loaf (page 234), heated ½ cup canned corn ½ cup canned button mushrooms Orange from allowance	309	12.3
Snack Remaining Fiber-Filler with milk from allowance 1 Fibermed Apple/Currant Biscuit	50	6.0
Total	**1,058**	**46.6**

1,000-Calorie Menu #9

	Calories	Fiber (g)
Daily allowance: Fiber-Filler, 1 cup skim milk, an orange, and an apple or pear	450	23.0
Breakfast Half portion of Fiber-Filler with milk from allowance Orange from allowance		
Lunch 1 portion Carrot and Lentil Soup (page 231) 4 whole-wheat crackers ½ medium banana	247	10.6
Evening meal 1 portion Beef and Bean Casserole (page 236) 1 cup cauliflower, cooked ½ cup green beans, cooked 1 portion Plum Charlotte (page 242)	358	13.0
Snack Remaining Fiber-Filler with milk from allowance Apple or pear from allowance		
Total	**1,055**	**46.6**

1,000-Calorie Menu #10

	Calories	Fiber (g)
Daily allowance: Fiber-Filler, 1 cup skim milk, an orange, and an apple or pear	450	23.0
Breakfast Half portion of Fiber-Filler with milk from allowance		
Lunch 1 Sardine and Tomato Pizza (page 235) Green salad: a few lettuce leaves, a few slices of cucumber, a few rings of green pepper, and 1 tablespoon oil-free French dressing Orange from allowance	299	7.4
Evening meal ½ chicken breast, all skin removed 1 portion Curry Sauce (page 229), thawed (Cover the chicken with the curry sauce and bake in a covered dish at 400°F for 45 minutes, or until the chicken is tender and cooked through.) ½ cup frozen peas, cooked Apple or pear from allowance	336	10.8
Snack Remaining Fiber-Filler with milk from allowance		
Total	**1,085**	**41.2**

1,250-Calorie Menu #1

	Calories	Fiber (g)
Daily allowance: Fiber-Filler, 1 cup skim milk, an orange, and an apple or pear	450	23.0
Breakfast Half portion of Fiber-Filler with milk from allowance 1 slice of whole-wheat bread, toasted and spread with 1 teaspoon diet margarine and 1 teaspoon honey or marmalade	101	1.2
Lunch 1 Sardine and Tomato Pizza (page 235) ½ cup shredded cabbage, mixed with 1 medium carrot (grated) and 1 tablespoon diet mayonnaise Apple or pear from allowance	330	8.0
Evening meal 1 portion Paprika Chicken (page 239) ½ cup mashed potatoes (with a little milk from allowance, no butter) ¾ cup cabbage, boiled Orange from allowance	361	12.7
Snack Remaining Fiber-Filler with milk from allowance 1 Fibermed Apple/Currant Biscuit	50	6.0
Total	**1,292**	**50.9**

1,250-Calorie Menu #2

	Calories	Fiber (g)
Daily allowance: Fiber-Filler, 1 cup skim milk, an orange, and an apple or pear	450	23.0
Breakfast Half portion of Fiber-Filler with milk from allowance 1 medium banana	85	2.7
Lunch 1 portion Carrot and Lentil Soup (page 231) 1 slice of whole-wheat bread, toasted and cut into fingers Apple or pear from allowance	198	8.8
Evening meal 1 (4-ounce) lean loin lamb chop, broiled 1 portion Barbecue Sauce (page 227), heated and served with lamb chop ¾ cup frozen mixed vegetables, cooked 1 portion Tutti-Frutti Ice Cream (page 244) served with orange from allowance, sectioned	573	14.5
Snack Remaining Fiber-Filler with milk from allowance		
Total	**1,306**	**49.0**

1,250-Calorie Menu #3

	Calories	Fiber (g)
Daily allowance: Fiber-Filler, 1 cup skim milk, an orange, and an apple or pear	450	23.0
Breakfast Half portion of Fiber-Filler with milk from allowance		
4 whole-wheat crackers, spread with 1 teaspoon diet margarine and 2 teaspoons honey or marmalade	120	1.6
Lunch 1 slice of whole-wheat bread, toasted and topped with 1 medium tomato (sliced) and 2 tablespoons grated Swiss cheese, heated under the broiler until cheese is melted		
Apple or pear from allowance	140	2.7
Evening meal 1 portion Beef and Bean Casserole (page 236)		
1 large baked potato		
12 Brussels sprouts, boiled		
1 portion Blueberry and Apple Crumble (page 245)	584	18.6
Snack Remaining Fiber-Filler with milk from allowance		
Orange from allowance		
Total	**1,294**	**45.9**

1,250-Calorie Menu #4

	Calories	Fiber (g)
Daily allowance: Fiber-Filler, 1 cup skim milk, an orange, and an apple or pear	450	23.0
Breakfast		
Half portion of Fiber-Filler with milk from allowance		
2 whole-wheat crackers, spread with 1 tablespoon low-calorie strawberry preserves	63	0.9
Lunch		
1 portion Corn Potage (page 232)		
1 (1-ounce) slice boiled ham, chopped (Heat the Corn Potage and sprinkle on the chopped ham.)		
1 slice of whole-wheat bread spread with 1 triangle Laughing Cow cheese		
Orange from allowance	353	7.1
Evening meal		
4 ounces cod, haddock fillet topped with 1 portion Tomato Sauce (page 226) and baked in oven at 350°F for 20 minutes, or until fish is done		
½ cup frozen peas, cooked		
1 cup cauliflower, cooked		
1 portion Tutti-Frutti Ice Cream (page 244) served with apple or pear from allowance, cored and sliced	398	17.0
Snack		
Remaining Fiber-Filler with milk from allowance		
1 Fibermed Apple/Currant Biscuit	50	6.0
Total	**1,314**	**54.0**

1,250-Calorie Menu #5

	Calories	Fiber (g)
Daily allowance: Fiber-Filler, 1 cup skim milk, an orange, and an apple or pear	450	23.0
Breakfast Half portion of Fiber-Filler with milk from allowance Orange from allowance		
Lunch 1 (3-ounce) hamburger, broiled and served with 1 portion Barbecue Sauce (page 227), heated ⅓ cup canned baked beans in tomato sauce Apple or pear from allowance	330	14.5
Evening meal 1 portion Pork with Prunes (page 238) ¾ cup cooked cabbage 1 portion Rhubarb and Bread Pudding (page 243) topped with ¼ cup vanilla ice cream	501	14.0
Snack Remaining Fiber-Filler with milk from allowance		
Total	**1,281**	**51.5**

1,250-Calorie Menu #6

	Calories	Fiber (g)
Daily allowance: Fiber-Filler, 1 cup skim milk, an orange, and an apple or pear	450	23
Breakfast Half portion of Fiber-Filler with milk from allowance		
Lunch 1 portion Zucchini and Corn Flan (page 233) Chopped lettuce 2 medium tomatoes Apple or pear from allowance 1 Fibermed Apple/Currant Biscuit	342	15
Evening meal 1 portion Chili con Carne (page 237) 1 cup cauliflower, cooked ½ cup green beans, cooked 1 portion Plum Charlotte (page 242) topped with ¼ cup vanilla ice cream	437	16
Snack Remaining Fiber-Filler with milk from allowance Orange from allowance		
Total	**1,229**	**54**

1,250-Calorie Menu #7

	Calories	Fiber (g)
Daily allowance: Fiber-Filler, 1 cup skim milk, an orange, and an apple or pear	450	23.0
Breakfast Half portion of Fiber-Filler with milk from allowance 1 medium banana	85	2.7
Lunch 1 portion Creamy Pea Soup (page 230) Cottage cheese sandwich: 2 slices of whole-wheat bread, 2 lettuce leaves, ¼ cup cottage cheese Orange from allowance	275	10.6
Evening meal 2 Jones pork dinner sausages served with 1 portion Sweet and Sour Sauce (page 228), heated ¾ cup cabbage, cooked ¾ cup canned corn Apple or pear from allowance	382	10.9
Snack Remaining Fiber-Filler with milk from allowance 1 Fibermed Apple/Currant Biscuit	50	6.0
Total	**1,242**	**53.2**

1,250-Calorie Menu #8

	Calories	Fiber (g)
Daily allowance: Fiber-Filler, 1 cup skim milk, an orange, and an apple or pear	450	23.0
Breakfast Half portion of Fiber-Filler with milk from allowance 1 egg, boiled 4 whole-wheat crackers, spread with 1 teaspoon diet margarine	158	1.6
Lunch 1 Sardine and Tomato Pizza (page 235) Chopped lettuce 2 tablespoons pickled beets Apple or pear from allowance	288	6.0
Evening meal 1 portion Lamb with Split Peas (page 240) 12 Brussels sprouts, cooked 1 portion Pear and Apricot Mousse (page 241)	421	10.7
Snack Remaining Fiber-Filler with milk from allowance Orange from allowance		
Total	**1,317**	**41.3**

1,250-Calorie Menu #9

	Calories	Fiber (g)
Daily allowance: Fiber-Filler, 1 cup skim milk, an orange, and an apple or pear	450	23.0
Breakfast Half portion of Fiber-Filler with milk from allowance		
1 slice of whole-wheat bread, toasted and spread with 1 teaspoon diet margarine	81	1.2
Lunch 1 portion Carrot and Lentil Soup (page 231)		
6 whole-wheat crackers		
Apple or pear from allowance	229	10.2
Evening meal 4 ounces calf's liver, sliced, brushed with 1 teaspoon oil, and broiled		
1 portion Sweet and Sour Sauce (page 228)		
½ cup Birds Eye Frozen Rice with Peas and Mushrooms, cooked without added butter		
¼ cup vanilla ice cream		
Orange from allowance	456	4.4
Snack Remaining Fiber-Filler with milk from allowance		
1 Fibermed Apple/Currant Biscuit	50	6.0
Total	**1,266**	**44.8**

1,250-Calorie Menu #10

	Calories	Fiber (g)
Daily allowance: Fiber-Filler, 1 cup skim milk, an orange, and an apple or pear	450	23.0
Breakfast Half portion of Fiber-Filler with milk from allowance		
1 medium banana	85	2.7
Lunch Shrimp sandwich: 2 slices of whole-wheat bread spread with 1 tablespoon diet mayonnaise and 2 tablespoons canned shrimp, topped with 1 tomato (sliced) and chopped lettuce		
Apple or pear from allowance	246	4.6
Evening meal 4 ounces cod or haddock steak, thawed and covered with 1 portion Curry Sauce (page 229) and baked in the oven in a covered dish at 375°F for 25 minutes, or until the fish is cooked through.		
1 cup canned button mushrooms 1 cup green beans, cooked 1 portion Blueberry and Apple Crumble (page 245)	546	21.4
Snack Remaining Fiber-Filler with milk from allowance Orange from allowance		
Total	**1,327**	**51.7**

Alcohol

Ideally, for fast weight loss and for improved health and fitness, it is better to avoid alcohol while following the F-Plan.

Realistically, however, if you feel deprived and miserable because you are not allowed any alcohol, you will not stay on the diet for long, so it is better to allow yourself a little. Obviously, in terms of calories you can afford to drink more alcohol at one time if you drink only occasionally, on the weekend, rather than every day.

Most women can lose weight very successfully on 1,250 calories a day, and some can even lose on 1,500 calories a day, while nearly all men will achieve a good weight loss on 1,500 calories a day. Most people can allow themselves a little alcohol while they are dieting, so long as they set aside 100, 200, or 250 calories for their drinks. This means that a woman who can lose weight on 1,250 or 1,500 calories a day and wants to include an alcoholic drink or two should choose a menu that provides 1,000 or 1,250 calories, thus allowing up to 250 calories for alcoholic drinks. Men should choose a menu of 1,250 to 1,300 calories daily and allow 200 to 250 calories for alcoholic drinks on those days when they know they will want a drink.

On the following pages you will find a calorie chart that will enable you to include drinks as part of your total diet.

ALCOHOLIC DRINKS CALORIE CHART

Aperitifs	*Calories*
per bar measure, 1½ ounces, 1 jigger	
Dubonnet red	170
Dubonnet white	108
Martini & Rossi vermouth,	
extra dry	143

Beer
 12-ounce can or bottle
Ale, mild   148
Beer, regular (Budweiser)   150
Beer, light   96

Cider, fermented, 6 ounces   71

Liqueurs
 1 cordial glass
Anisette   65
Apricot brandy   67
Benedictine   70
Crème de Menthe   67
Curaçao   55
Kirsch   65
Tia Maria   70

Port and sherry
Port, muscatel, 1 wineglass   158
Sherry, cream, 1 sherry glass   95
Sherry, medium, 1 sherry glass   84
Sherry, dry, 1 wineglass   85

Spirits
 per bar measure, 1 jigger, 1½ ounces
Whiskey, gin, vodka, rum, 40 proof   110

Wine
 4 fluid ounces
Red, sweet   169
Red, dry   73
Rosé   120
White, sweet   85
White, dry   65

Champagne, 1 wineglass   85

Nonalcoholic Drinks Calorie Chart

	Calories
Chocolate drinks	
Cocoa, 1 tablespoon	58
Chocolate syrup, 1 teaspoon	18
Malted milk powder, 1 teaspoon	27
Ovaltine, 1 teaspoon	30
Fruit juice (½ cup)	
Apple	60
Grape	60
Orange	56
Pineapple (canned, sweetened)	64
Tomato	24
Milk (1 cup)	
Whole	150
2%	137
Skim	90
Reconstituted from nonfat dry powder	125
Sodas and mixers	
All diet sodas: Diet Shasta, Tab, Diet Pepsi, etc., 1 can (12 ounces)	1
Bitter lemon, 8 ounces	128
Club soda	0
Coca-Cola, 1 can	144
Ginger ale, 8 ounces	90
Lemonade, 1 cup	90
Orange soda, 1 can	167
Pepsi, 1 can	156
Tonic, 8 ounces	88

Index